Back to strength:
a manual for back care

Life is bad for backs – make your back good for life

This book is dedicated to all back pain suffers.

Back to strength:
a manual for back care

By

Christina Folliard

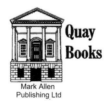

Quay
Books

Mark Allen
Publishing Ltd

Quay Books Division, Mark Allen Publishing Group, Jesses Farm, Snow Hill,
Dinton, Nr Salisbury, Wilts, SP3 5HN

© Mark Allen Publishing Group Ltd, 1998

British Library Cataloguing-in-Publication Data
A catalogue record for this book is available from the British Library

ISBN 1 85642 091 4

Printed in the UK by Redwood Books, Trowbridge, Wilts

Contents

Acknowledgements

I would like to thank all the students I have worked with over many years as I have developed my ideas for back care and the programmes to alleviate back pain. I would especially like to thank my daughter, Gaby, for all her love and support, and my son Tom for the inspiration. And finally thanks to Tamzin Ewers for helping to edit the manuscript.

Introduction

During a normal day, without warning, a slight movement can send your back into spasm, racking your body with pain. It is an unbearable, intense pain — unlike any pain you have experienced before. You are now one of the back pain statistics you have read about:*80% of the population suffer with back pain at some time*; *more working days are lost because of back pain than any other physical ailment.*This now that includes you.

Panic is about to take over your rational mind as you try to remember what you should do to alleviate the pain. Advice floods in from friends, family, shopkeepers, paperboys/girls, anyone who can see you are in pain because of the strange way you are walking. A helpful friend will comment that when their back went a warm bath sorted it out. Whereas another friend will recommend ice packs and bed rest.

All the advice you receive suggests that instant relief will come from a variety of remedies — rest, exercise, painkillers, a strong Scotch, herbs, oils. For every piece of advice, there will be a contradiction. Your head is spinning. Your temper is now short. Your breathing is increasing and the pain does not go away. It feels as if it is going to be with you for the rest of your life. What are you going to do?

This book will give you a course of action, both for the immediate and the longterm to avoid a recurrence of the problem. The book examines the back, the causes of back pain, posture, relaxation techniques and the benefits of exercise.

The main focus of the book is a series of exercises that not only help to alleviate back pain but also strengthen the back. The exercises are easy to follow. These are followed by exercise plans that work both in the short and the longterm. Prevention is better than cure, so if you do not have a back problem use this book to keep your back strong and problem-free. This book will give safe, sensible advice, examining the entire problem.

Sufferers of back pain see themselves as passive victims of pain, often being told by the medical profession, and others, that they must live with it or that it is unavoidable normal wear and tear.

This book will challenge that attitude. It will allow victims of the back pain to take control of their bodies. Control will not come overnight. There is no instant, easy answer, Remember that if you do nothing, in a few months the pain will return, to your life again.

You must decide now — are going to sort out your body, working to produce a body that will cope with the demands you make of it, without giving way to back pain? This book will give you a safe plan to develop back strength and show how to keep your back and, indeed, your whole body strong and flexible. You probably look after your home or your car better than you look after your back; now is the time to change that attitude. Decide to develop a strong, healthy back and enjoy a pain-free life — and go back to strength.

As with any exercise programme it is advisable to check with your GP. before you begin the exercises. However, because holistic approach of thes courses, I am sure that your GP. will be pleased that you are taking steps to help yourself and control your back problem. Note: Throughout this book the term 'back' includes the spine.

Section 1
Aspects of back care

This section examines:

- Understanding your back
- Area of importance for maintaining back strength
- Posture
- Causes of back pain
- Action plan for immediate relief from back pain
- Learning to relax
- Breathing techniques

Understanding your back

In order to control the problem that causes your back pain you need to have a basic understanding of the anatomy of the back. You need to understand the structure of the spine, the relationship between the spine and the muscles and nerves, and how the spinal system works. This knowledge will explain why you have a problem. More importantly, it will explain the action you are about to take to live free from back trouble permanently. This simple outline is essential reading to provide the terminology used throughout the book.

The spine

The spine is a series of curves (see *Figure 1.1*). These curves enable the vertebral column to aborb the shocks of daily life. Anything that pulls the curves out of shape weakens the back and makes it vulnerable to damage. Therefore it is extremely important to retain these curves as you work with your body.

What is a spine?

The spine consists of 24 individual bones called vertebra, although there are occasionally 25 vertebra. The vertebra are stacked on top of each other, like children's building bricks. Balancing at the top is the head and, at the base is the pelvis. Each of these blocks, or vertebra, link together to form a continuous moveable, flexible column. The spinal cord is enclosed within the vertebral column. It consists of nerve cells and bundles of nerves connecting all parts of the body with the brain. It is through the nerves that pain is transmitted. The spinal cord varies in length between 16" and 18" (42-45 cm.) in an adult. It extends from the base of the brain in the skull to the beginning of the lumbar vertebra. Below this a bundle of nerve roots descends down the vertebral column until they reach their respective openings. This bundle is called the *cauda equine* because it resembles a horse's tail.

Although they are alike, the vertebra are different in ways that will enable you to move in every direction using different part of the spine. This very difference also contributes to the weak areas in the spinal column.

Figure 1.1: The spine

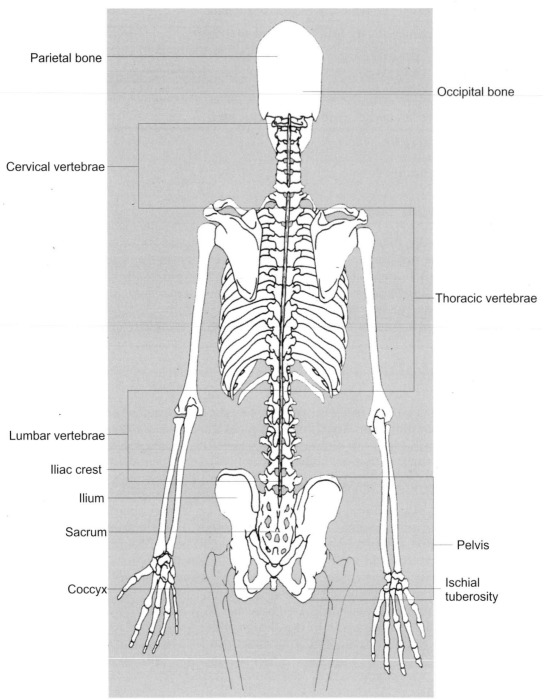

There are three types of vertebra: cervical; thoracic and lumbar. The position of which are illustrated in *Figure 1.1*.

Cervical vertebrae

These vertebra are in the neck and hold the head in a balanced position and allow the head to move in many directions. They are smaller vertebra than the next group.

Thoracic vertebrae

These are are situated in the chest region and attachment the spine to the ribs, while the ribs protect the organs of the chest by forming a cage. These vertebra allow the body to twist as well as bend.

Lumbar vertebrae

These are situated in the lower back. They begin to transfer the weight of the body into the pelvis; also from the legs into the body. The lumbar vertebra allow the body to bend

Intervertebral discs

These are plates of fibrocartilage that connect any two adjacent vertebrae. They give the spine flexibility. They act as shock absorbers, protecting the brain and spinal cord from the impact produced by running and other movements. They look like liquorice allsorts, and move in a similar fashion when squeezed.

Discs are vulnerable to twisting forces that rupture the fibrous outer coat allowing the pulpy inner material to protrude causing painful pressure on the adjoining nerves. This condition is often called a 'slipped disc', but it would be more correctly described as a 'disc protrusion' or 'disc hernia'.

Nerves

The vertebrae form a continuous channel and the spinal cord is enclosed within this channel. Nerves emerge through holes in the vertebrae. These nerves go to every part of the body and relay messages to and from the brain. Abnormal pressure on nerves will result in pain. The nervous system controls and integrates all body movements and functions. The importance of the nerves can be seen in *Figure 1.2* which illustrates how the nerves feed the major organs of the body. Therefore, a strong, healthy back will be beneficial to numerous other aspects of well-being.

Figure 1.2: Nerves leaving the spine, feeding the major organs of the body

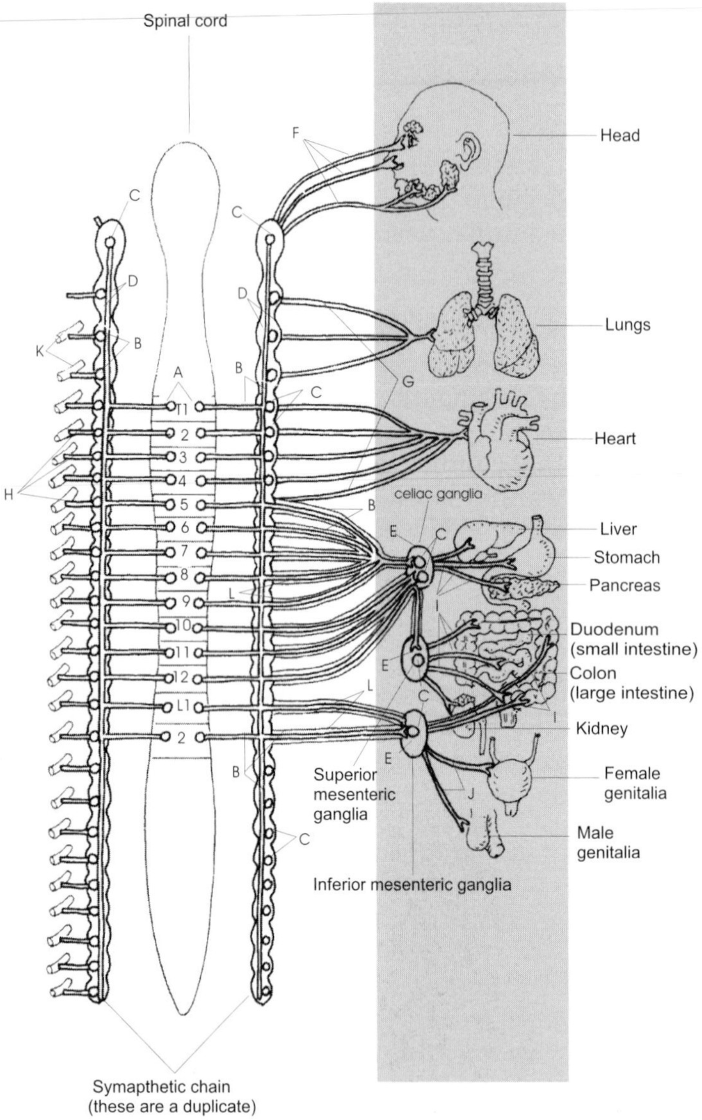

Figure 1.2 illustrates how the nervous system is structured in terms of the spine. It shows where the nerves leave the spine and which organs they feed.

Key
Preganglionic neurones
A   Cell bodies
B   Axons
Postganglionic neurons
C   Cell bodies
D   Point where these axons to the thoracic viscera leave the spine
E   Prevertebral ganglion which is made up of three major sets of cell bodies
F   Axons to the head and neck
G   Axons to the thoracic viscera
H   Axons to the skin which feed the sweat glands, arrector pili and blood vessels
I   Axons to the abdominal viscera
J   Axons to the pelvis and perineum
K   Spinal nerves
L   Examples of splanchnic nerves

The pelvis

One of the most important structures of the body, the pelvis transfers the upper body weight into the legs. It gives stability, strength, and flexibility to the body, and aids articulation. The pelvis consists of two hip bones, the sacrumand the coccyx. This forms a bony ring and two joints, called the sacroiliac joints. These joints suffer many problems as a result of poor posture and lack of exercise.

The spinal column enters the pelvis at the sacrum, and the transfer of weight occurs here. The back was not designed for 20th century living.

The sacrum

Sacrum consists of five vertebrae fused together in the shape of a triangle. Attached to the last vertebra of the sacrum is the coccyx. This is a small triangular bone, formed by three to five fused vertebrae. It is believed to be the last vestige of a prehistoric tail.

Figure 1.3: The pelvis showing the sacroiliac joints

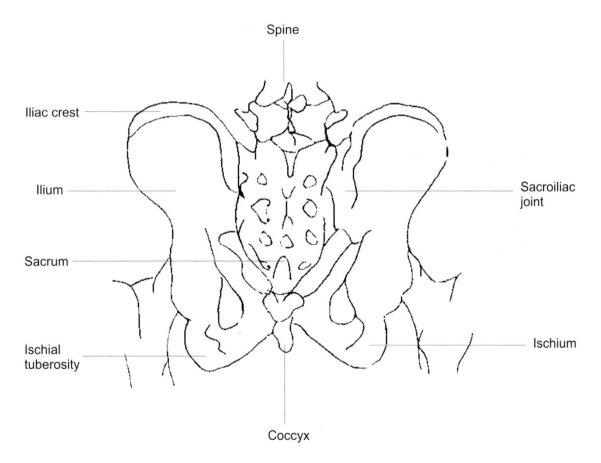

Joints

A joint is where two bones meet. There are various types, with different functions. Joints are usually classified by their movement or structure. The spine contains, many joints. The joints under discussion are the synovial joints. These are moveable joints.

Flexion is bending forward. Therefore the flexor muscles curl. (see *Figure 1.4a*).

Extension means to stretch. Therefore the extensor muscles allow the body to stretch upwards (see *Figure 1.4b*).

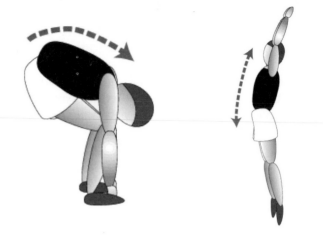

Figure 1.4a: Flexion   **Figure 1.4b:Extension**

Muscles

Muscles for speed (see *Figure 1.5a*) and for movement (see *Figure 1.5b*).

Figure 1.5a: Speed   **Figure 1.5b: Movement**

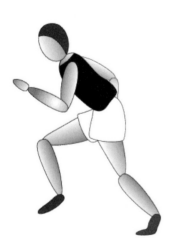
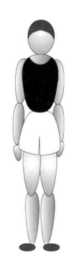
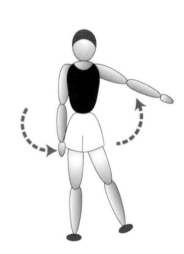

Muscles give stability and support to the bones and organs

They work in pairs to produce movement. Joints need both sets of muscles to produce movement. Muscles do not work in isolation. They involve other muscles from the same and other areas of the body. Therefore, it is important when improving back strength not to work only on strengthening the obvious areas. The entire body needs work. Exercises need to be designed for the whole body. (see *Figures 1.6* and *1.7*).

Often muscles are not equal on both sides, though they should be. Muscles are affected by poor posture, stress, poor diet and incorrect exercise. Years of misuse will result in a body that is suffering from unbalanced muscle groups.

The relationship of the entire muscle structure of the body is often forgotten. Headaches and migraine can be the response of the body to a pelvic misplacement or coccyx that has been damaged after a fall. A shoulder problem may occur because of a low back weakness, and knee problems because of pelvic rotation. Any imbalance in posture will have an effect, either higher or lower in the muscle structure, leaving those areas vulnerable to damage.

Muscles are joined to bones by tendons; these are tough bands of fibre that stretch when movement is produced. Ligaments are tough bands of fibre that hold the joints in place like elastic bands.

Tendons and ligaments do not easily repair and require regular movement to stay supple. Exercise will prevent them stiffening or slackening. Ligaments scar after injury and it is difficult to restore them to their original condition. They also have a limited blood supply, and must be exercised regularly to maintain their nourishment. Whiplash is a common ligament injury. Ligament strain can often be felt after prolonged sitting, especially if one is sitting incorrectly.

Muscular tension

Muscles are never entirely free from tension. The muscles retain 'tone' even when resting. Muscular tension is affected by mental attitudes such as anger, worry, fear and sadness. Any stress will have an adverse effect on muscles and, therefore, on back stability. This is a very important part in the re-education of your body as you work towards strengthening your back.

Figure 1.6: Simple muscles — anterior

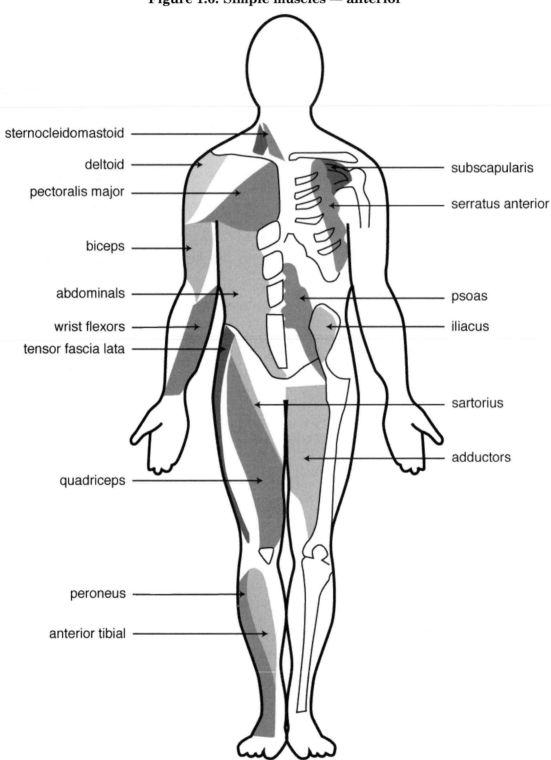

sternocleidomastoid

deltoid

pectoralis major

biceps

abdominals

wrist flexors

tensor fascia lata

subscapularis

serratus anterior

psoas

iliacus

sartorius

adductors

quadriceps

peroneus

anterior tibial

Figure 1.7: Simple muscles — posterior

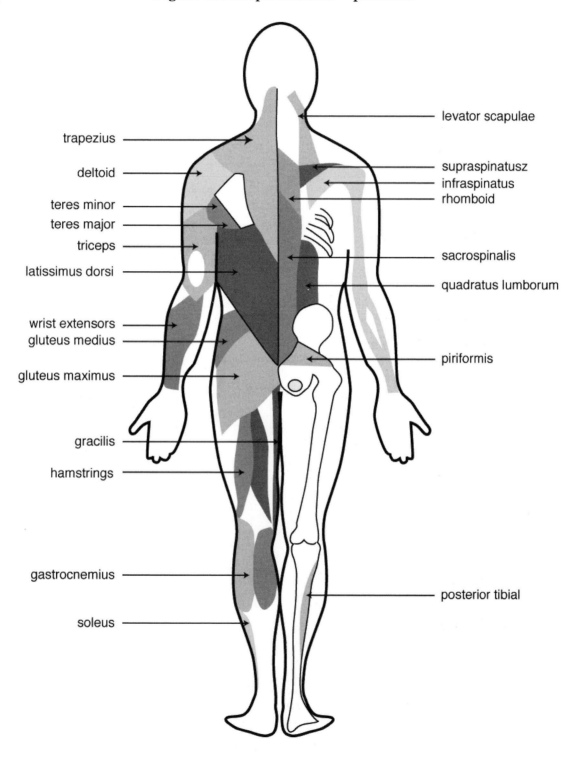

trapezius

deltoid

teres minor

teres major

triceps

latissimus dorsi

wrist extensors

gluteus medius

gluteus maximus

gracilis

hamstrings

gastrocnemius

soleus

levator scapulae

supraspinatusz

infraspinatus

rhomboid

sacrospinalis

quadratus lumborum

piriformis

posterior tibial

Areas of importance for maintaining back strength

Pelvic girdle

The weight of the head, the upper limbs, and the upper body (including organs) is transmitted to the legs through the pelvis. In addition, shocks and movement felt by the legs are transmitted into the body via the pelvis. The pelvic crossroads are extremely important in maintaining a pain-free back. As I have mentioned before, the pelvis and sacroiliac joints were not designed for 20th century life. The environment inflicts stresses and strains on this area of the body as never before. This is a major factor in the increase in back problems over the last few decades.

Sacroiliac joint

To keep the pelvis strong and flexible, you must also look higher, to the abdomen, and lower, to the legs. If these areas are not doing their work of support correctly, the pelvis and back will suffer, and low back pain the result. Leg muscles are often used incorrectly , with the result that they give insufficient support to the pelvis.

Abdominal area

There are superficial and deep muscles in the abdominal area; all are very important in maintaining back strength, and must be exercised correctly.

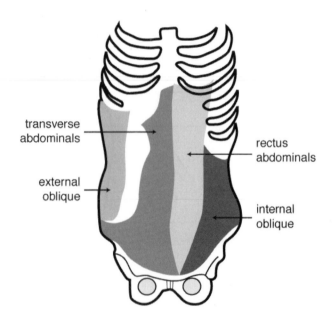

Figure 1.8: Abdominal muscles

Legs

The legs also have many muscles associated with back strength and stability, and need to be exercised correctly and on a regular basis to ensure a trouble-free back. See *Figures 1.4* and *1.5* for anterior and posterior views of the muscles in the legs.

Posture

Bad posture is responsible for 80% of back problems. Good posture can prevent this statistic. What is bad posture? Why should it affect the back so much? What is good posture and how can it affect the back? This section will answer those questions, giving you an insight into another possible cause of your back problem. Incorrect posture will affect the muscular structure of the body. Muscles on both sides of the body should be equal in strength and flexibility, giving support to the joints. Incorrect use of your body will result in your body having one side that is dominant in strength and flexibility, while the other side will be weak and therefore vulnerable to damage. This one-sidedness can occur when you constantly cross the legs, stand badly, sit slumped in a chair or work with the body angled to the same side. These examples and many more instances will let your muscles become unbalanced, long and flexible on one side, while short and tight on the other. You need to be vigilant with your posture until correct posture becomes a habit.

You must gain an understanding of your body through correct posture work, just as a good driver understands the car through driving. Your body, over the years, will have become badly co-ordinated. This will be mainly due to incorrectly performed movements. It leads to uneven muscle tension. Poise and correct posture have become outdated words in the English language, just as back problems have become common.

We will look at what bad posture is, and exactly why it causes pain, stress, fatigue and ill-health. How to deal with it? I think you will be surprised.

If you think about good posture it would be useful to re-read the paragraphs on the spine. Remember that the spine is a series of curves that must be maintained to remain pain-free.

There is an incorrect belief, that tucking the tail under, or tilting the pelvis under, is good for the back, and is the correct way to stand. Nothing could be further from the truth. Indeed, if practiced too often, it will give you a back problem. This tucking-in of the pelvis will instantly give you a flatter stomach, which while maybe highly desirable, is dangerous as it makes backs vulnerable. Flat stomachs can be achieved through diet, correct posture and exercise, not by tucking the bottom under.

What are the causes of bad posture?

Bad habits are formed through lazy use of the body. Here are a few examples to start you thinking about your own posture.

Leisure activities

Watching television slumped at an angle, always in the same chair and therefore slumped to the same side. Watching lying on the floor, propped up by the arms.

Driving

Sitting at an incorrect angle, without sufficient support in the lumbar curve. Remember, cars are designed for the average back. Are you average? Check you have sufficient support as you drive. Watch for shoulder tension. Use the breathing techniques to breath away road rage.

Work

Sitting, standing or twisting for too long all weaken the back. Try to move around every half hour. Practice spinal flexibility exercises in your lunch break. Drink a lot of water.

Sports

One-sided sports, for example tennis, which overdevelop the dominant side of the body can cause back problems if the other side is not exercised as well. Try to warm up with the other hand. Sports played only at the weekend can also do more harm than good if incorrect stretching is used to prepare the body. Swimming can be useful as an exercise to increase flexibility. However, unless the strokes are performed correctly, the result can be backache. Breast stroke and free-style can cause neck and low back problems. Keep your head in the water as you do breast stroke. Change stroke every ten minutes.

Sleeping

Mattresses that have lost their ability to support the body should be changed. Take advice from a bed specialist. Turn your mattress regularly, side to side as well as top to bottom. Check your pillow height is correct, giving sufficient support for the head to be in the correct position. Sleeping in the recovery position will weaken a strong back. Try lying in this position on the floor and see how it twists your pelvis and back. Use pillows as support.

Walking

Walking is extremely good for the body, especially when the posture is correct. Do not wear shoes with high heels, and check that trainers do not have too much heel height, as thick heels when used for walking will tighten leg muscles. Watch the angle of your head. Remember to think: *stand tall, walk tall*.

Sitting

Slumped without any support in the lumbar area, sitting with the legs tucked up to one side or sitting with crossed legs: these are all habits designed to weaken the back. Tell your hairdresser or dentist if you have a back problem, and sit accordingly.

Look at everything you do, and review your posture; any action that is repeated becomes a habit and has the potential to weaken the body. We tend to be habitual people, always parking the car in the same way, answering the telephone with the same hand. Habits can cause back problems. If you think about your posture in daily life you will probably be able to make adjustments that will be beneficial for your back.

Think about your posture as much as you can. Ask yourself: *Am I stretched comfortably? Is my neck relaxed?*

Once you begin to change your habits from bad to good, you will be horrified at how you have abused your body through bad posture. Remember the statistic and do not allow yourself to become one of the number.

Correct posture can make the body look slimmer and feel better. As you grow older, the once-upright body loses suppleness and movements become less easy and more set which, in turn, gives you a less energy-efficient body with back vulnerability and constant tiredness. This consequence does not have to happen. You can prevent this occurring. It is never too late to change your habits and regain a comfortable, supple body that is strong and flexible; a body you can be proud of. One way to prevent that situation is to improve your posture and strengthen your back through using the *Back to strength* programme.

Causes of back pain

There are numerous causes of back pain, some of which are listed below.

Accidents

Any kind of accident can affect the back, from a car accident to tripping over a kerb. It is the sudden movement that sends the muscles into spasm. It is important to have a supple and flexible back so that it can easily absorb the bumps and knocks which occur throughout life.

Beds

Your mattress may be the source of your back pain. It is important that it gives you correct support. Check with a bed specialist how long your bed should be used for.

Sleeping

An incorrect sleeping position can cause or aggravate a back problem. During sleep muscles relax and this allows the joints to be pushed or pulled without the correct support. We are creatures of habit, especially when sleeping. We tend to curl up on the same side night after night. This leaves the back vulnerable. Use pillows to support the body during sleep and try to establish new sleeping patterns.

Pregnancy

Hormones released during the early months of pregnancy soften ligaments. This may leave the spine unstable and unable to cope with the extra weight. This will leave the lower back vulnerable to discomfort and pain. Gentle exercise will help to protect the spine.

Birth and after

A difficult labour can leave the pelvis misaligned. You should have your back checked by a chiropractor or osteopath to avoid problems later. As the baby gains weight it is necessary to carry the child correctly so that there is no undue strain on your back. A child should be carried either at the front or back of your body and not on one hip. Begin your exercises as soon as your doctor agrees and ensure you exercise every day. It is important to make time for yourself as well as your baby.

Cars

Manufacturers of cars are now well aware of the importance of correct, supportive seating so that both driver and passengers are in ergonomically designed seats. However do check that your car gives the support your back requires. After all your back is individual and your car is not. Use a rolled up hand towel to give you the extra support where it is needed.

Chairs

Check that all the chairs you use are helping your back remain strong. Ensure that you sit straight at your work station and not at an angle. Again, use a rolled up hand towel to give the necessary support. Whenever you sit on a chair think about your back. For example, suggest to your hairdresser you use a forward basin when they wash your hair as a 'backwash' may aggravate either a neck or back problem.

Environment

In the past few decades our way of life has drastically changed. People sit for hours in cars, at desks or at machinery. They work with their hands and eyes rather than their whole body. Twentieth century technology, with the emphasis on cutting down on physical work, has been disastrous for the body especially the back. Try to use your body whenever possible, use the stairs not the lift or walk to the shops. There ire endless ways to increase your physical activity.

Genetic

Back problems may be inherited, for example scoliosis (a lateral curvature of the spine), kyphosis or lordosis (excessive curvatures of the spine), leg length difference. These problems and many others can be helped with the help of gentle exercise.

Hot baths

Relaxing in a hot bath may seem like a good idea but it could do more harm than good because you lie in the shape of the bath, which allows the natural spinal curves to pull out of the correct position as the muscles relax in the hot water.

Illness

Any physical problem that your body has to cope with will affect your back. Even a simple cold may re-start an old back problem. Tension and pain will affect your muscles, introducing muscle spasm and nerve pain. Even if you do not feel very well try to do some gentle exercises along with relaxation exercises and breathing practice. Do not wait for a problem to start, protect your back and prepare against pain.

Incorrect exercise

Exercise routines must include a warm up period and a cooling down period, especially if the exercises are strenuous and aerobic. Introduce exercise into your life carefully and effortlessly. Discomfort should not be the result of exercising.

Lack of exercise

Lack of exercise will weaken your muscles and you will lose a great deal of flexibility, leaving your back vulnerable to daily living. However busy and full your life is, this cannot be a substitute for back exercises; rushing around all day is not the same as an exercise roputine. Find time to exercise and save your back from pain.

Leisure activities

Some types of activitity may aggravate an existing imbalance in your muscle groups. Ensure that your hobbies use your body correctly. Gardening should be carried out with care. For example, bend correctly when weeding; lean on one knee rather than both.

Sport

In sports that favour one side (golf, tennis, bowls) the less used side must be warmed up equally by stretching and exercising. Swimming is extremely beneficial for increasing strength and flexibility. However, you should vary the type of stroke; do not use breaststroke too much. Swim correctly with the head in the water.

Menstruation

Pre-menstrual syndrome may affect your back for up to ten day before menstruation as well as during it.

Muscle imbalance

Muscle imbalance occurs slowly and inperceptably, and can become a long-standing problem. Constantly using the body more on one side will leave one set of muscles stronger and more flexible, and the other remains weaker and shorter. This type of imbalance puts the back at risk. Uneven support is often a major problem for back pain sufferers. Try to use both hands equally for manual work.

Overweight

Excess weight overloads the joints, especially in the lower back area and the knees. As you lose weight it is important to begin the exercises gently and slowly in order to strengthen these vulnerable areas .

Underweight

Being underweight can cause problems when weak muscle leaves the back with insufficient support and strength. Fast growing teenagers, especially boys, are often vulnerable to back pain. Slouching and carrying school bags on one shoulder when experiencing a growth spurt can be the beginning of intense pain in the lower back.

Stress

Stress will attack the most vulnerable parts of your body, tightening and knoting your muscles. If you have a history of back problems any stress in your life will cause the pain to return. Controlling your back pain means controlling the stress in your life. Use the relaxation plan and do your exercises carefully. Work with the gentle plan and take extra care with your posture.

The mind

The mind controls your response to any situation that you percieve as difficult. The mind will tighten muscles as tension sets in to your body, attacking the weakest part of your back. When life becomes stressful take extra care of your back. Be strong-minded about your daily exercises. Try to be positive and relaxed. Negativity effects the muscles badly; it is important to work with the relaxation plan.

Work

Any work that repeats an action will allow the muscles to develop in an unbalanced manner. It is essential to take regular breaks and constantly think about posture. Exercise daily to build up the strength and flexibility of the whole body.

The list is endless — think about your own case. Most of the problems above can be linked to bad posture.

Action plan for immediate relief from back pain

Identifying the problem

What causes pain to shoot through your back, and the muscles to go into a tight unyielding knot called muscle spasm?

A displaced bone is one of the main causes. This will cause pressure on nerves in the area of damage, and the muscles will tighten around the area in an effort to prevent further pain. Paradoxically, this results in a greater problem of muscular spasm and pain.

For so long the body will protect areas of vulnerability, allowing you to carry on with slightly displaced bones, held incorrectly by unbalanced muscles. This will go on and on, giving you an occasional twinge of pain and discomfort, or pain that goes away after a while. Your body accepts this misuse until, one day, it will say NO MORE with the result being an acute bout of pain that will not go away. So what are you going to do? Who do you ask to help?

Your first attack of back pain

If you have experienced this pain before, you will probably be aware of your physical limitations and the precautions that are necessary. But, if this is your first attack, you should consult your doctor. If you have unrelenting pain, tingling pains or pins and needles in any limb, loss of feeling in limbs, or a change in bladder or bowel habits, you MUST consult your doctor.

Action plan

1. Take arnica homeopathic remedy, preferably strength 30, though arnica 6 will suffice. Use hypericum if you have fallen on your coccyx. Homeopathy is a great help when treating back pain, and arnica tablets will help the body recover from the shock of an attack of back pain. Seek advice from a registered homeopath for a more personalised prescription.

2. Rub into the area of pain, and on the opposite side of the body, a muscle relaxant balm or an aromatherapy oil, which you can buy from health stores. You can also mix your own oils.

   Using an aromatherapy oil will help release the muscular spasm. Rub the oil gently into the muscles. Do not forget to rub oil into the opposite side to relax the overworked muscles. If you would like to mix your own oil, use some of the following essential oils. Remember, do not rub an essential oil directly on to the skin; it must be diluted in a vegetable oil. Sweet almond oil is very good. Other oils include:

   - Thyme

   - Roman camomile

   - Lavender

- Ginger

- Rosemary

- Marjoram.

If you want to mix your own, I recommend that you mix:

10 drops Rosemary

10 drops Marjoram

10 drops Lavender

10 drops Roman camomile

then dilute in 30ml of Sweet Almond oil.

Note: Do not use any of these oils (except lavender) if you are pregnant or you might be pregnant.

3. Rest for short periods, lying on your back with your knees bent. Support your head to relax your neck and place a small towel in the lumbar area. Place pillows under the legs to release tension in the pelvic area.
   If you have a prolapsed disc, rest is important and you must take your doctor's advice. However, too much rest can aggravate other back problems. When resting for reasonable lengths of time, it is important to rest correctly. Lying down will take the pressure off joints and muscles. Try not to drive or sit for periods of longer than 20 minutes without taking a break from your sitting position. Gently moving the spine and back muscles regularly, if sitting for long periods, is imperative. Do not carry medium weight objects, such as a young child. Lie in one of the following positions and work with a breathing exercise. Use a towel to support the lumbar area wherever you sit.

4. Work through your breathing exercise.

   It is important to do a breathing exercise during a back pain attack. This will help the muscles relax and release their spasm. It will also help to cleanse the body of the toxins that are a residue of stress and pain. Work through the breathing exercises, lying down, and try to repeat them every two hours. Concentrate on your area of pain or discomfort, breath into that area and, as you exhale, feel the pain going out with the breath, disappearing as you exhale. Inhale, take in a healing breath, into the same area, again releasing with the exhalation. Remember: exhalation relaxes the body.

5. Take pain killers, if necessary and acceptable to you. Take care not to injury the body when the pain has been relieved. You still have a back problem it has just been camouflaged and is in potential danger of further damage.

6. Very, very gentle exercise.

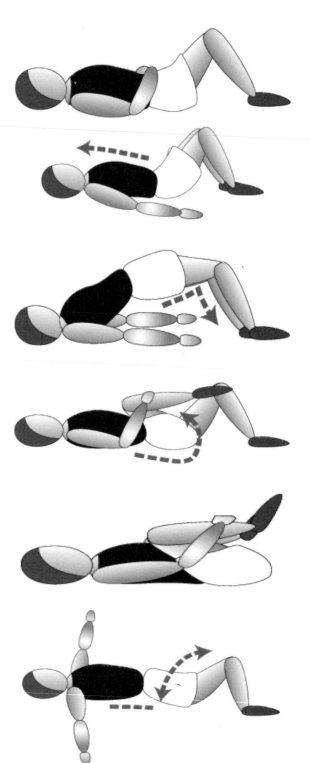

- Lying on your back, take twelve breaths. Hands on the abdomen, support back where necessary.

- Tilt the pelvis — imagine you are pulling the pubic bone towards your face. This will flatten the low back to the floor. Pause for three seconds, then release. Repeat several times.

- Lying on the back with the knees slightly apart, feet by the buttocks. Very gently, lift your bottom off the floor as you inhale. Then return to the floor as you exhale. Take two breaths. Repeat for as long as it does not hurt.

- Lying on the back as before, bring one knee towards the face, hold with the hands. Pause for one second and then replace the leg to the original position. Repeat with the other leg.

- Lying on the back, bring both knees on to the chest, or towards the chest. Gently support the knees with the hands and hold for six breaths.

- Lying on the back with the knees bent, arms out to the side of the body. Gently allow the knees to go to one side of the body, towards the floor. Bring them back up and go to the other side. The movement should be gentle and relaxing, not painful.

- Bring the knees on to the chest and gently ease them towards the body.

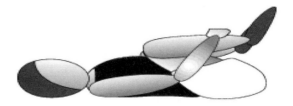

- Lying on the floor with the knees bent. Place the hands on the abdomen and breath gently, as if down to the hands. Stay for 6–12 breaths.

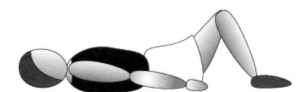

7. Relaxation techniques — direct your mind to the pain.

   See the section on relaxation techniques. Dab lavender oil on the temples. Drink camomile tea sweetened with honey, not sugar.

8. Use ice packs

   Wrap a pack of frozen peas in a towel. Apply for 20 minutes to the area of pain. Repeat as necessary. Ice sprays are available from the chemist.

9. Apply hot water bottle on muscles only . Do not place the bottle directly on to the spine or any area near it.
   Warmth from a hot water bottles can help relax a muscular spasm. Do not take baths, especially hot ones.

10. Relax as you move. Try to lift out of the pain without becoming tense in other areas. Moving the body will cause pain. However, staying in the same position can make the situation worse. Try to keep straight; ask a friend to look at your posture as you stand still and walk. Lift the body out of the pelvis to keep the weight evenly distributed. Whenever you sit down, make sure that the lumbar curve is supported. Take a small hand towel in your pocket or bag, and use it always, especially when sitting for periods of longer than 10 minutes. When getting dressed avoid standing on one leg as you put on your clothes; sit or lie down to put on socks or tights and shoes.

11. Drink a lot of water.

12. Use lavender oil to help relax.

13. Try to be confident that you are going to control the pain.

What now?

After a few days, you will begin to feel better and the pain will be easier. Now is the time to take action to prevent further trouble. Your back pain will return if you do nothing except carry on with your way of life not changing the habits that caused the problem in the first place. Decide now that you are going to prevent your back becoming a major restraint in how you live your life. Constantly thinking: *I can not do this, my back will not stand it* is not living life to the full. Positive action and a little self-discipline will change your body and your life.

Make an appointment with an osteopath or chiropractor, to ensure your bones are in their correct position. This will enable you to be free from nerve pain and the resulting muscle spasm.

There are many excellent books written by chiropractors, osteopaths or physiotherapists on the subject of manipulation. This is a self-help book. The emphasis is on you.

Learn to relax — break the circle of stress

Do you understand what stress is, and what the word 'stress' means? How stress transfers into back ache and pain?

> stress = tension = backache = tension = stress

Unnecessary stress and tension are a major hurdle in the treatment of back problems. Identifying stress can be extremely difficult, as we all delude ourselves one way or another. One important aspect to remember is that what is stress for one person is not a problem for another. One person's stress is another person's challenge or, as the proverb states: *one man's meat is another man's poison*. Do not underestimate what may cause stress to you.

What is stress?

The environment is perceived differently by each individual. For example, my daughter plays loud pop music in her extremely untidy bedroom to relax. For her, it is peaceful, sitting among the debris of many weeks. For me, it is stressful. It makes me tense and irrational to have to cope with her bedroom and the noise!

Here are a few examples of what could be deemed stressful situations to make you think and smile. I am sure you can think of a few of your own.

Routine	Music	Punctuality	Challenges	Unemployment
Lateness	Driving	Other drivers	Road rage	Work
Health	Money	Christmas	Hot Weather	Cold weather
D.I.Y	Holidays	Noise	Birthdays	Travel
Outings	Relatives	Cars	Videos	Animals
Television	Untidiness	Addictions	...	...

Remember, anything that upsets you causes frustration or anger. The response will be within your physical body, allowing it to become vulnerable to an attack of back pain. Therefore it is important to focus upon controlling the stress in your life.

How to control stress

There are two main options:

- Emigrate

- Cope with your stress.

The first is not very sensible, for eventually your stress will follow you and therefore build up wherever you live.

The second option is far more practical. You need to find ways to cope with your stress. Think about how stress makes you feel. It probably causes tension.

What is tension?

It is the physical response to any stressful situation, as perceived by an individual. Tension has a weakening effect on the body, especially the muscles, with the usual result of another bout of back pain for no apparent, comprehensible reason. Therefore, it is extremely important when you feel you are facing a stressful situation to take extra care with your back and the weak areas such as the neck, the low back and the knees.

The best method of controlling stress and tension is in a natural way.

Breathing techniques

breath control = mind control = no stress reaction

The may seem like a simple answer. So simple you are probably thinking *oh yes!* However, breath control is not a simple answer, as you are about to find out. Control will not come easily unless you work at it seriously.

The mind affects the breath and the posture is a simple statement that must be examined. Watch the body language of a happy person, then compare it with the body language of a stressed supermarket shopper, or of drivers trapped in a traffic jam. Be aware of the contrasting body language. The mind—body—breath link is important. So, what do you do about it? By reaching an understanding of breathing you will learn to think about your breathing and therby learn how to control your breath.

To understand your breath you must understand the mechanism of breathing.

The breath

The breath consists of four parts. Each part has a different effect on the mind and, therefore, the body. And you thought you just breathed in and out:

- Inhalation — stimulates the mind

- Pause — contains the stimulation

- Exhalation — relaxes the mind

- Pause — enhances the relaxation.

Watch the breathing pattern of various people, friends, family. A good example of breathing patterns is a contestant in a quiz show on the television. If the contestant has a run of difficult questions the breathing pattern will be shallow and fast; as the questions become easier, the breathing will relax.

This response is important. You must recognise the link between stress and quick, shallow breathing. The body works this way naturally, and you can learn to control it. Remember:

stress = quick, shallow breathing

Also remember, it is impossible to experience stress and retain a slow relaxed breath.

Your breathing rate, the number of breaths you take per minute, will vary according to age and physical health. But the stress will still influence your breath length (Inhalation and exhalation count as one breath). A variety of breathing rates are illustrated in *Table 1.1*.

Table 1.1: Breathing pattern in an average adult (35–65 years, male or female)	
stressed	25–50 breaths per minute
normal	10–16 breaths per minute
relaxed	5–10 breaths per minute
controlled	3–5 breaths per minute
very relaxed	2–3 breaths per minute

Remember, your breathing rate is as individual as you are.

How to develop and control your breath

Aims:

- To understand your breath, and the effects stress has on your breath, with the cumulative affect on the body

- To gain control of your breathing, naturally and permanently, in order to relax your muscles at will

Precautions:

- Do not strain the breath

- Do not become light-headed or breathless

- Do not hold the breath in an attempt to lengthen the breath

- Control must be achieved naturally, at your own pace

Equipment required:

- Ticking clock

- Straight-backed chair

- Pillow or cushion

- 2 or 3 paperback books

Practice aims

- To count how many breaths you take in five minutes

- To count how many seconds it takes you to inhale and exhale over a period of time

- To increase the length of time and still keep the mind quiet

- To try and decrease the number of breaths taken by increasing the breath length and using your lungs to full capacity.

Posture for breathing practice

Sit in an upright chair, with feet under legs so that thighs are parallel to the floor. The shoulders should be relaxed, hands on the lap, relaxed, head not pulled forward, lumbar area supported with a towel.

If sitting is not comfortable, practice breathing lying down with the head supported on paperback books so that the chin is tucked in and feels comfortable. The lumbar curve should be supported, and the legs supported with pillows. Hands should be relaxed on the abdomen. But breathing will be easier sitting, allowing the ribs to move fully. The body, in either position, must be comfortable, so that the mind is not disturbed by physical discomfort during the breathing practice.

Beginning the breathing practice

1.   Make sure you feel comfortable.

2.   Close your eyes.

3.   Be aware of your breathing, your body. How are your ribs moving? Which way are they moving?

4.   Begin to count your breath, using a ticking clock to regulate your counting. Count in seconds.

5. Do not give up. Your mind is insistent. It will begin to distract you and tell you this is silly, pointless. It is not. It is extremely important in your *Back to Strength* back care plan. So do not give up.

6. When ready, begin to count your breath for five minutes, and record the number of breaths taken. Remember that one breath is both inhalation and exhalation.

7. Keep a record of the number of complete breaths taken.

8. Try to practice breathing correctly during the day, when you are involved in different activities.

9. Once you can breathe properly, you can begin to develop the breath and use it to control muscle spasm pain by relaxing the muscles.

10. Practice using the breath to relax specific areas of the body. For example, as you inhale, concentrate on your right side between pelvis and rib cage. Breath out, tell yourself to relax, release that area, and feel any unnecessary tension leaving that area. Try the shoulders now. However, it is important when you begin to concentrate on an area not to tighten it before you relax it. While this may be unconventional advice, many years' experience of working with stressed patients has convinced me that first tightening an area of tension does not achieve its release. Practice releasing areas of your body to experience the control your mind and breath have over the muscles.

11. At the end of your breathing practice, think positively about your back. Reassure yourself that you are now in control of your back problem, and that your back problem is not controlling your life.

12. Decide on an 'affirmation' about your back and repeat it at the end of your breathing practice and at various times during the day. Do not underestimate the power of positive thought. One possible affirmation is:

    My back is becoming stronger and I am now in control it.

    Spend a little time developing an affirmation you are comfortable with.

Learning about your breath, gaining control over it and understanding the strength of mind is an important part of back care. This is the essential art of *Back to Strength*. Everyone experiences difficulty when first listening to the breath. The mind is like a radio that is constantly switched on. Be patient, it will come. Control is not easy.

Also remember the following pages are examples only. Do not try to copy them. Find your own breathing level.

Breathing practice record

Keep a record of your breathing practice so that you can see your own development. An example of such a record is illustrated in *Table 1.2*.

Table 1.2: Example of a breathing practice record				
Day	Monday 9.30	Tuesday 9.30	Wednesday 19.30	Thursday 20.00
Time taken	5 minutes	5 minutes	5 minutes	5 minutes
Number of breaths taken	30	30	28	28
Number of seconds of inhalation		5		6
Number of seconds of exhalation		8		10

This record reveals longer breath and a more relaxed mind on Wednesday and Thursday. This could be due to the time of day, or relief that work is over.

Carry on recording your breath lengths, until you can see how your breath changes according to your mental and physical state. Once you feel comfortable with this concept, it is time to develop and control all parts of your breath, so you can use it effectively when your life is stressful and a threat to your back.

Remember, after the inhalation and exhalation there is a pause, a recoil, as the body prepares to draw in a new breath or release an old one. This recoil requires very gentle development and it is essential that you do not strain the body or breath in an attempt to lengthen it. Allow the recoil to lengthen, be aware when the body wishes to breathe again. Your breath should become slower and deeper. This must be a natural development, otherwise it will desert you in times of need.

Record your breathing rate as before. Remember, a breathing rate is a highly individual ratio that can not be compared with anyone else's, only your own. Trying to compare breathing rates is as pointless as if everyone were trying to wear size 5 shoes.

Table 1.3: Example of an extended breathing practice		
Day	Monday 9.30	Tuesday 9.30
Time in minutes	5	5
Number of breaths	16–17	25–30
Number of seconds of inhalation	6	4
Number of seconds for a pause	2	1
Number of seconds of exhalation	8	6
Number of seconds for a pause	2	2

The ratio of breathing in *Table 1.3* shows that on Monday the complete breath was more relaxed, therefore the mind and body were more relaxed, reducing the back's vulnerability.

Remember, do not strain or hold the breath at any time. It takes a long time to stress your body with tension, and it may take a long time to relax it. Try to gradually increase the time you spend at your breathing practice 15 minutes a day is ideal. Keep the attention on counting at all times. Remember, everyone will experience difficulty in keeping the mind clear, not just you.

Especially if you suffer from high blood pressure, heart problems, or eye pressure problems, you take care not to hold or strain the breath.

Section 2

Exercises

This section includes:

- The benefit of exercise

- The approach to exercise

- Beginning to exercise

- Breathing techniques

- Exercises

- Beginning the exercise programmes.

The benefit of exercise

Why should you exercise?

It has been shown that underuse of muscles either before or following a back injury can turn an acute attack into a chronic problem. A short-term problem will become a long-term problem which leaves the back constantly vulnerable to pain.

Physical changes take place in muscles when they are underused. These changes affect the muscles' function, leaving the back weak and susceptible to muscle spasm and prolonged back pain. This is why it is essential to do exercises specifically designed to keep the back strong. Many exercises are irrelevant for this purpose, and indeed some exercises can do more harm than good. The exercise programmes in this book have been developed following years of research and work with patients recovering from acute back injury as well as patients with long-term problems.

Although the exercise plan appears to be simple it is essential to take things very slowly. Do not be in a hurry to progress. Once you begin to exercise, strength and suppleness will slowly develop. It is important that you do not shock your body into more spasm.

The exercise programmes must be practised every day of every week of every year. Many patients claim that they do not have enough time to exercise every day. Others are under the impression that because they are on the go all day they do not need to exercise.

But remember: if you do not make back exercises a part of your daily routine, you are leaving yourself vulnerable for back trouble to reappear.

What do you want to achieve by doing exercises? A strong back with as little effort as possible? A body that will stand up to the demands of your busy life? To feel confident in your back's ability to cope with anything you have to do? Focus upon this.

These exercises, once learnt, will take only 15 minutes in your day. As the day contains 24 hours, can you really say you cannot find 15 minutes in your day to provide your back with the strength it deserves? You must include exercise into the daily routine of body care: washing; cleaning teeth; shaving or make-up; exercise. It is as easy as that to make exercise a part of your daily routine.

It has been found that when an exercise programme is schedualed into a morning routine, it will still be part of that routine a year later. However, when the intention is to find time during the day, very soon one day's exercises are missed, then two days', then it is the slippery slope of intermittent exercising and the liklihood that the pain will return.

You should approach back strengthening exercises with caution and awareness. Be aware that, once your back begins to regain strength and suppleness (this timescale will vary between individuals), if you do not continue to exercise and build up your strength, your back will become even more vulnerable to strain. While you enjoy your re-found flexibility it will quickly disappear if you do not continue to exercise.

The approach to exercise

It is important to bear the following points in mind when thinking about exercise:

1. Approach exercise with care and attention. Learn to appreciate the effect it is having on your body.

2. Exercise with awareness of the specific area you are trying to stretch; concentrate on movement in that area.

3. Do not approach your exercise courses and plans with the attitude: *I have to get this done.* Enjoy them, they are your friends.

4. Exercise using the breathing techniques to assist you, so that if the pattern of your breath changes, for example it becomes shorter or faster than your usual breathing pattern, stop the exercise. Look at what you were doing. A change in the breath shows you were over-extending your body, making it vulnerable to strain. The exercise may be too strenuous for your body at the present time. Use breathing to mirror your body's response to the exercises. Are they in harmony with your body? Is your breathing quiet?

5. Be aware that your body changes daily. What was comfortable yesterday may be too demanding today. There are many factors to consider when practising, for example you may be more flexible in warm weather. The day of the week may have an effect on your body. Think of the 'thank goodness it's Friday' feeling against the 'Monday morning' feeling. That will translate

into your muscles. All of these and more will have an effect on your body and you will need to exercise accordingly. Use breathing to ascertain your true mental state before you begin to exercise. That is why you should always take time to lengthen the breath and listen to it before you begin. Six to eight breaths are enough.

6. Learn to distinguish between stretching and pulling the muscles. Stretching feels comfortable and easy. Pulling does not.

7. Be aware of the difference between work and damage.

8. Do not cause yourself pain, ever.

9. If you have recently had a cold, or any lowering ailment, take extra care.

10. Women should take extra care with back exercises a week before and during menstruation.

11. If in any doubt, consult your GP.

12. Do not be in a hurry to progress through the courses. While they seem very gentle in the beginning, it is essential to awaken your muscles slowly, without causing damage. Then you can develop a strong, supple body fit for life.

13. Do continue to work with your breathing practise. Once you are aware of your breathing you do not need to record it. As you progress you will begin to understand how it responds to your stress levels and you can adjust it accordingly.

14. The speed at which you develop depends on many factors, especially how weak your muscles have become through misuse.

Beginning to exercise — awaken your muscles to a new life

Notes to read before you attempt this exercise programme

1. Slow, rhythmical movements are essential. Do not work the exercises quickly, even if you are in a hurry.

2. Keep attention on the areas that are marked. If you do not feel the work going into that area, stop, re-read the details of the exercise and try again. If you still do not feel it in the specific area, modify as suggested until the work is felt correctly.

3. Stretch slowly with the breath, release as you breathe out.

4. Do not provoke pain. Stop if you do.

5. Use the breath with every movement. This is essential.

6. Slow control of your body should be your aim.

7. When working with asymmetrical (one-sided) exercises, work your weaker side last. Work into the weakness with the breath and really concentrate on the work area.

8. Modify the exercises if any cause discomfort to your weak area. For example, in standing exercises, do not take the arms above the head but raise them gently, therefore *Figure 2.1* becomes *Figure 2.1a*.

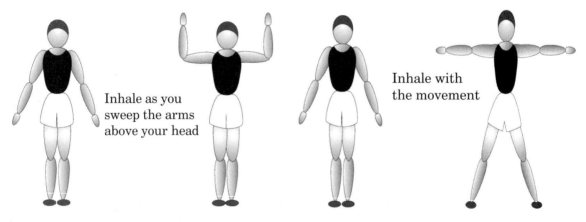

Inhale as you sweep the arms above your head

Inhale with the movement

Figure 2.1   **Figure 2.1a**

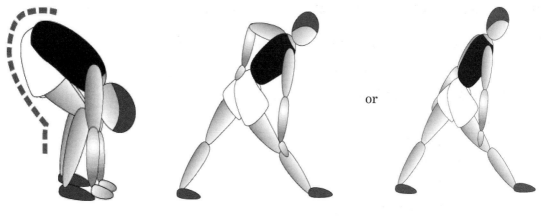

or

Figure 2.2   **Figure 2.2a**

Or you could modify a side movement as in *Figure 2.2* to *Figure 2.2a*. Remember that bending the knees will release too much work in standing exercises protecting the lower back.

9   Be aware that your mind is cunning and will try to avoid using the weak areas in your body. The body will make use of other areas to help weak muscles. Through your slow work using the breath, you will be aware that this is happening.

10.   Follow the instructions carefully to avoid working the body incorrectly.

For example abdominals that are weak may not exercise correctly. As you lift the head and shoulders off the floor, the lower back should go to the floor as the abdominals tighten and work (see *Figure 2.3*).

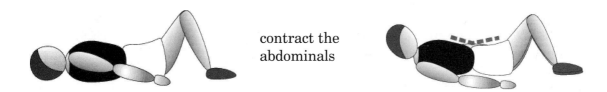

contract the abdominals

Figure 2.3

However, what may happen is that the head and neck do the work instead of the abdominals; the mind will convince you that the work is going into the abdominal area when all you are doing is possibly damaging the neck area.

What should you do? Be very aware of the abdominal area before you begin. Tighten the muscles and try to use that movement, for example the tightening of the abdomen, to lift the shoulders up, using the minimum of lift. Less exhertion will actually achieve more. You can modify the exercise by putting the hands behind the neck and giving the neck and head support.

Another example is the squat. Keep the back straight, heels on the ground, knees apart (see *Figure 2.4.*). What actually happens is that the body leans forward and the knees pull apart and the heels come off the ground (see *Figure 2.4a*). The way to modify the exercise is to do less work by barely bending the knees and keeping the back straight. This modification will work the body harder, therefore gradually developing the muscles until you are strong enough to go further into the exercise but remember to do so safely (see *Figure 2.4b*).

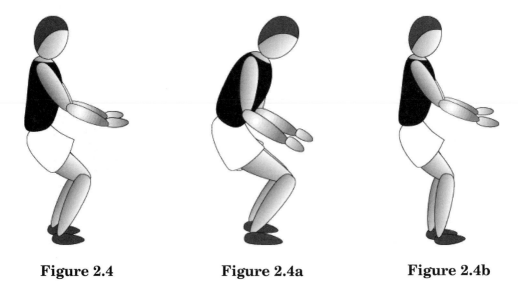

| **Figure 2.4** | **Figure 2.4a** | **Figure 2.4b** |

11. Relax as you go into a movement, give your body a chance to work with the exercise.

12. Repeat the exercises as many times as you feel comfortable with it. Sometimes once is sufficient; then you can try to build up to six or eight repetitions.

13. Occasionally in the modifications, the breathing sequence may change from the rule, for example breathe in as you move out and open the body. This is to allow the body to develop gently, progressing towards a final exercise. To modify an exercise means to adapt it for your own needs, both physically and

mentally. It is an important part of this exercise programme and one of the reasons the *Back to Strength* course works.

14. Pauses between exercises and take a few breaths. Do not rush from one exercise into the next. Allow your body and mind to return to normal before asking them to work on the next exercise. Pause for up to six breaths between exercises.

Breathing techniques

How to use the breath with the exercises

Breath in when you move the body away from the mid- or straight line of the body. Opening up the body indicates an inhalation.

If you are standing, raise the arms above the head, inhale as you move the arms upward (see *Figure 2.5*).

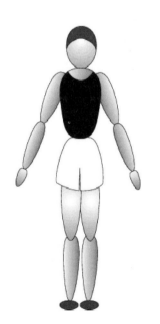
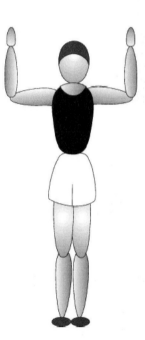

Inhale as you sweep the arms above the head

Figure 2.5

Or if lying on the floor inhale as you move the arms above the head (*Figure 2.6*).

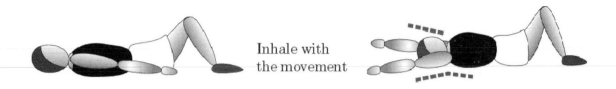

Inhale with
the movement

Figure 2.6

Or lie on your back and lift the bottom off the floor and as you do so inhale (*Figure 2.7*).

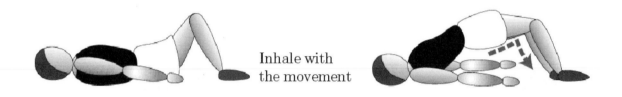

Inhale with
the movement

Figure 2.7

Breathing out, or exhaling, occurs as you close the body down. Therefore in the standing position you exhale as you lower the arms from above the head (see *Figure 2.8*).

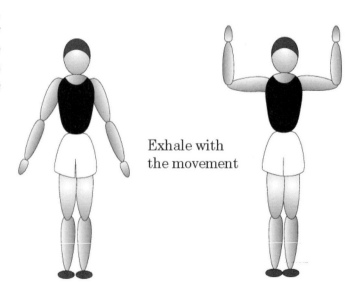

Exhale with
the movement

Figure 2.8

Or if you are lying on the floor exhale as you move your arms back to your sides (see *Figure 2.9*).

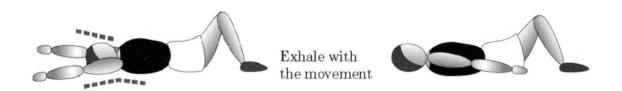

Exhale with
the movement

Figure 2.9

Or exhale when you lower your bottom (see *Figure 2.10*).

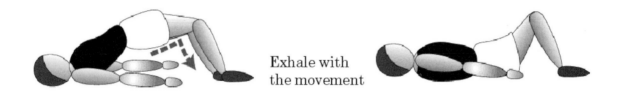

Exhale with
the movement

Figure 2.10

This gives you a complete movement with the breathing as illustrated in *Figure 2.11*.

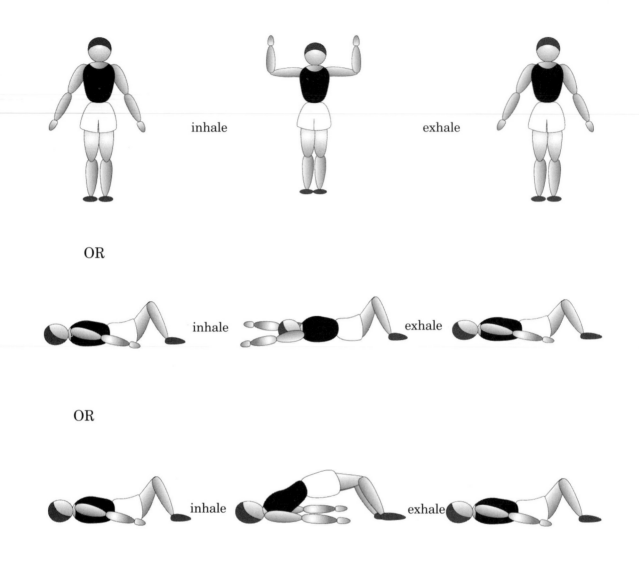

inhale   exhale

OR

inhale   exhale

OR

inhale   exhale

Figure 2.11

It is essential to work this way to gain the full benefit from the programme of back strengthening. Keep reminding yourself of the breathing pattern until it becomes natural to move with the breath when you exercise.

Exercises

Instructions on how to work with the exercises correctly. Read them carefully and take note of the breathing sequence.

1. Lying on the floor with the knees bent, with the feet comfortably away from the bottom, knees slightly apart, hands relaxed on the abdomen. If necessary, support the head with paperback books and the legs with a pillow. This is the starting position for most of the supine exercises, also for the breathing practise. Do not attempt to flatten the back to the floor.

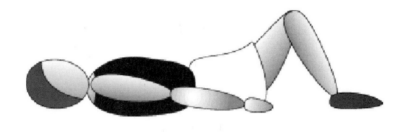

or

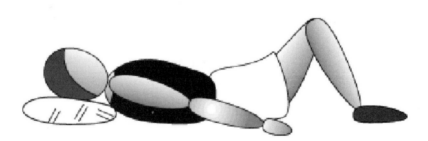

Exercise 1

2. Lying on the floor with knees bent. As you inhale, move arms above head, resting on the floor behind the head if possible. Return on exhale, remembering not to overstretch arms.

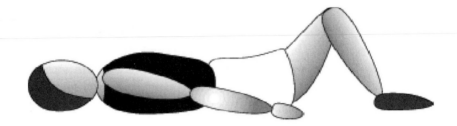

Inhale as you sweep the
arms above your head

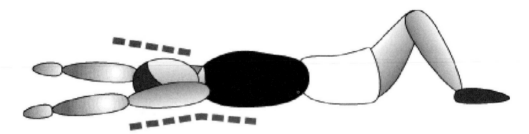

Exhale as the arms
return to your side

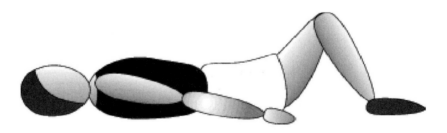

Exercise 2

3.   Lying on the back, slowly stretch one leg along the floor, pointing the toes away from the face. Return to original position as you exhale. Repeat with the other leg.

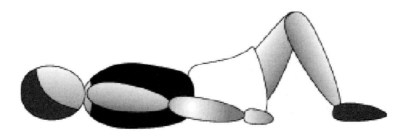

Inhale as you
straighten the leg

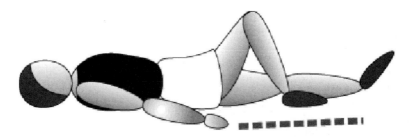

Exhale as you return the
leg to the starting position

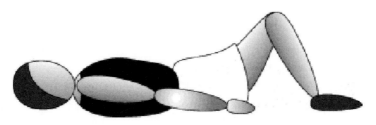

Exercise 3

4. Lying on the floor, knees bent. Exhale as you bring one leg towards the chest. Gently hold it with the hands. Then return leg to the original position as you inhale. Repeat with the other leg.

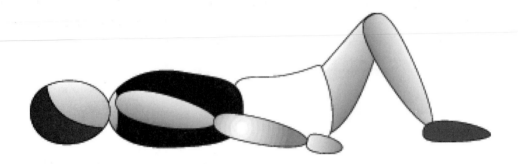

Exhale as the leg
moves into the chest

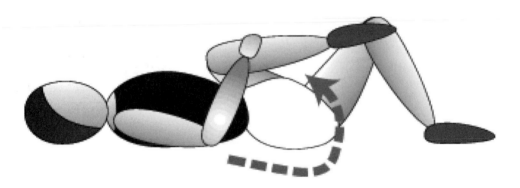

Inhale as the leg returns
to the starting position

Exercise 4

5. This exercise can be slowly developed as your body becomes stronger and the hamstrings become more flexible. Do not attempt the final movements until you can work with the modifications easily, without discomfort.
   Lying on the back, knees bent. Stretch one leg away, making one slow movement. As you inhale, bend the knee on to the chest and straighten the leg up towards the ceiling. This is performed as one action with one breath. Return the leg in the same way. Repeat with the other leg.

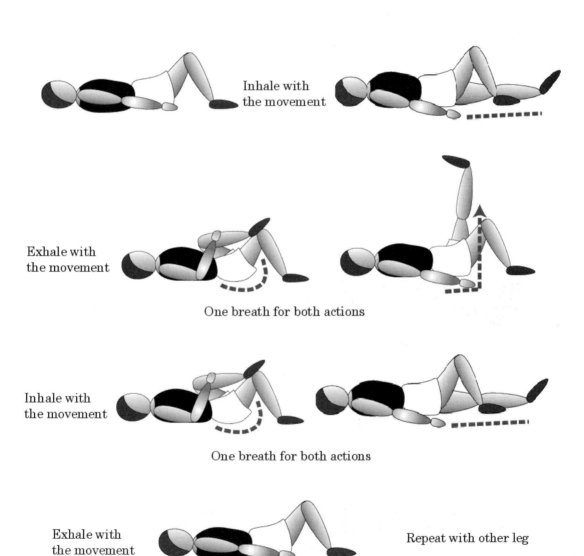

Inhale with the movement

Exhale with the movement

One breath for both actions

Inhale with the movement

One breath for both actions

Exhale with the movement

Repeat with other leg

Exercise 5

5a. Develop and extend exercise.

Lying on the back, stretch one leg out as you inhale. Exhaling, raise the foot towards the ceiling. As you inhale, point the toes towards the face. Exhaling, lower the leg to the floor. Inhaling, replace leg. It is important to move the leg towards the ceiling and return it to the floor on the exhalation. This affords the lumbar area the maximum safety during this demanding exercise.

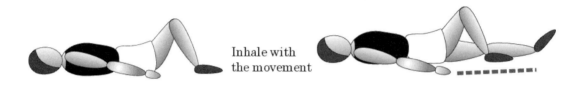

Inhale with the movement

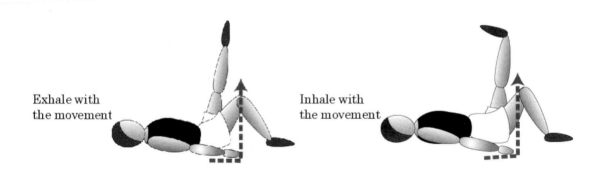

Exhale with the movement

Inhale with the movement

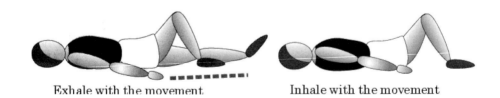

Exhale with the movement

Inhale with the movement

Exercise 5a

6. Lying on the back in the start postition, inhaling, allow one knee to lower to the floor. Exhaling, return leg to the start position. Repeat with the other leg.

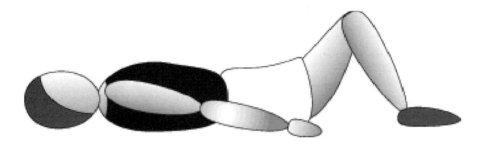

Inhale with the movement

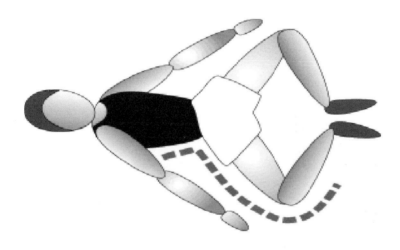

Exhale with the movement

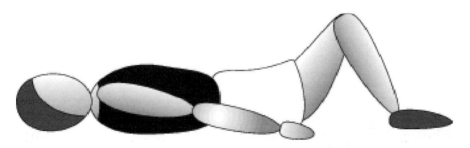

Exercise 6

7. Lying on the back, knees bent. As you inhale, lift the bottom off the floor. Exhale as you lower it back to the floor. Eventually you will be able to create an arch. However, to begin with just lift as high as you feel comfortable with.

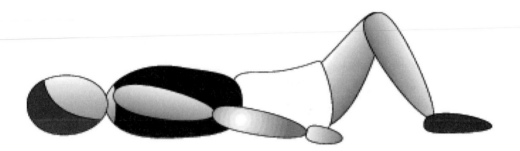

Inhale with the movement

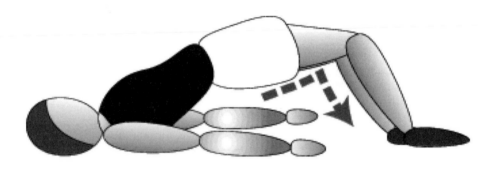

Exhale with the movement

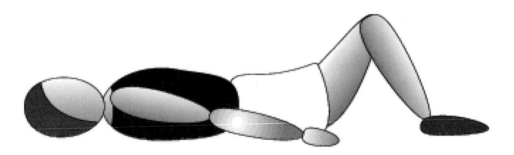

Exercise 7

7a. The same as above, this time take the arms above the head and relax them on the floor behind the head as you lift the bottom off the floor. Move your arms back to the side as you lower the bottom to complete the exercise. Inhale as you lift the bottom and arms up, exhale as you lower them back to the floor.

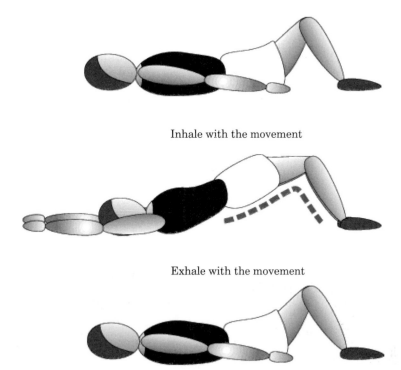

Inhale with the movement

Exhale with the movement

Exercise 7a

8. Lying twist. Lying on the back with the knees bent, arms relaxed to the side of the body, palms facing upwards. Exhaling, allow the knees to go first to one side of the body, then the other. Inhale when you return the legs to the centre.

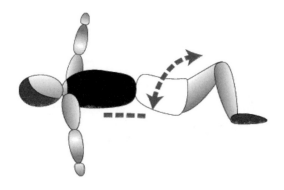

Exercise 8

9.   This is an excellent exercise to relax the back, although performed incorrectly it will add tension to the back.Use pillows under the knees if the floor is too hard for your knees. Work with the exercise until you can feel all parts of the back working, then add the breath to enhance the exercise. It is important to keep the shoulders relaxed and as much weight out of the hands as possible. The mind will try all kinds of ways to avoid working with tight, unsupple areas in the back. Try to work with the eyes closed and imagine that you have a stack of dominoes along your spine, lying from the tail to the head. As you move from one position to the other, imagine they are toppling over. Start on your hands and knees. Exhale as you raise the back so that it forms a gentle arch. Inhale as you return to the starting position. Exhale as you raise your back again. Inhale as you lower the back and curl the spine into the floor. Finally exhale as pull your bottom approximately 10 inches towards the feet. This is an important exercise for releasing tension. It must be performed correctly. practise until you can move all parts of the spine.You can modify the general position of Exercise 9 for arthritic hands or wrists so that you are resting on your elbows and forearms (see Exercise 9a).

This exercise is often incorrectly described as illustrated in *Figure 2.12*. This is not recommended. It is important not to allow the back to hollow too much as this puts the vulnerable joint L5S1 at great risk.

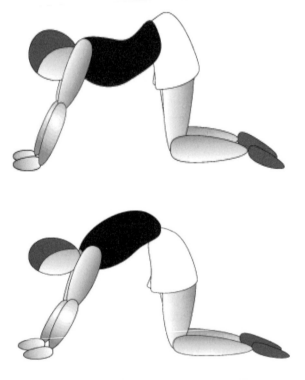

Figure 2.12: not recommended

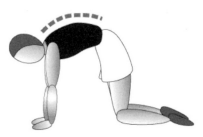

Exhale as you
move your back
towards the ceiling

Inhale as you
return to the
starting position

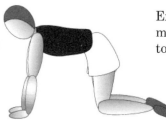

Exhale as you
move your back
towards the ceiling

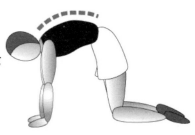

Inhale as you
gently lower the
stomach towards
the floor

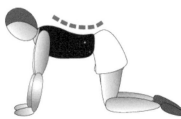

Exhale as you
move the bottom
towards the feet

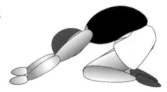

Exercise 9

Modify Exercise 9 by resting on your forearms instead of your hands

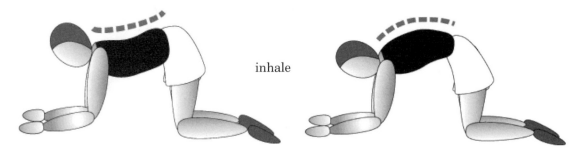

inhale

Exercise 9a

10. Sit on the heels with the shoulders relaxed, head held correctly and the hands relaxed on the lap as in figure A. Modify for varicose veins or troublesome knees by putting a pillow under the bottom and/or the knees as in figure B. Do not slump in the chest area. Be aware of the spinal curves and work with gentle, deep breathing.

Starting position as seen in A or use the cushion as in B

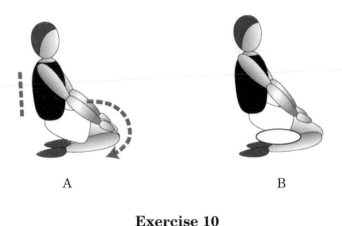

A   B

Exercise 10

11. Sit on heels, modify if necessary, back straight but not tensed. Inhale, move into a seated position, lowering the arms as you exhale. Keep the shoulders relaxed throughout the exercise.

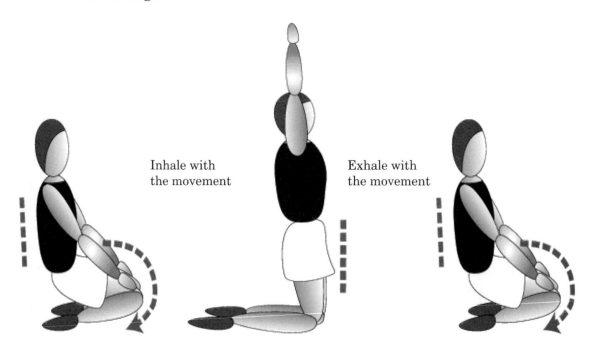

Inhale with the movement

Exhale with the movement

Exercise 11

12. Use a chair to bend forward on to, until you are supple enough to practise without one. Start in a seated, kneeling position with one arm tucked behind you. Keep relaxed in the waist area. Inhale as you rise to a kneeling position. Exhaling, go forward taking the straight arm on to the seat of the chair. Inhale, come back up to a kneeling position. Sit back on the heels. Take a breath before you repeat. Work the other side in the same manner, with one arm tucked behind the body. Keep the shoulders relaxed.

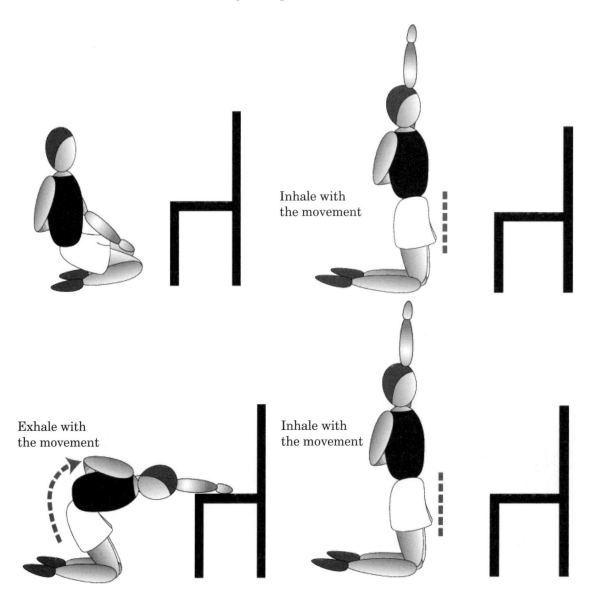

Exercise 12

13. Start in a seated, kneeling position. Inhaling, rise to a kneeling position with both arms above the head. Exhaling, bend forward, sweeping the arms sideways on to the back as you bend. Inhaling, return to a kneeling position, sweeping the arms sideways as you do so. Try to make as wide a circle as possible with the arms. Relax into a seated position as you exhale.

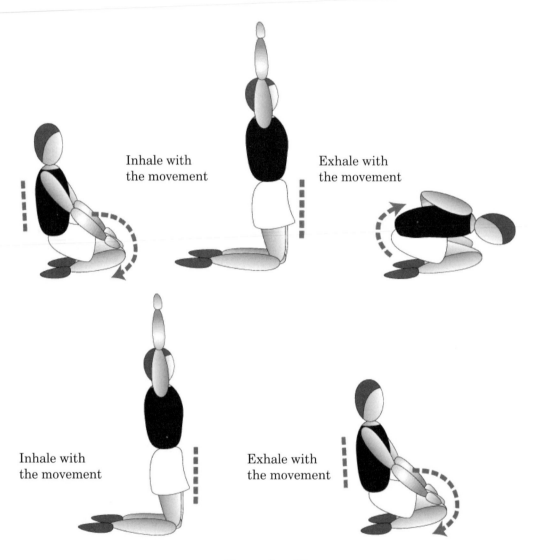

Exercise 13

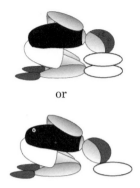

Figure 2.13

Exercise 13 can be modified for the not-so-supple by the use of books for the head to rest on (see *Figure 2.13*). Remove the books as you regain suppleness and strength.

14. Position yourself with the hands under the shoulders, the arms straight, the knees comfortably under the pelvis, slightly apart, the shoulders and back relaxed. Breath in and, as you breath out, lift the knees off the floor raising the bottom. Gently push the heels towards the floor, stretching the hamstrings. Return by bending the knees and slowly returning them to the floor. At first this will be difficult and the heels will remain a long way from the floor. However, as the muscles gradually stretch and you regain suppleness, it will become easier.

   Note: If you suffer from high blood pressure, heart problems or eye disorders, or have recently had a respiratory infection, take great care with this exercise.

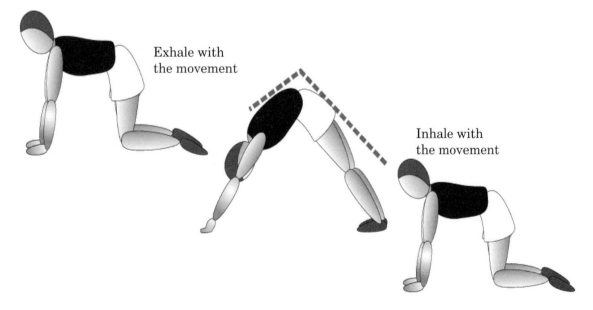

Exhale with the movement

Inhale with the movement

Exercise 14

15. Remain in the position below to relax the body after breathing work is very beneficial. Modify with paperback books.

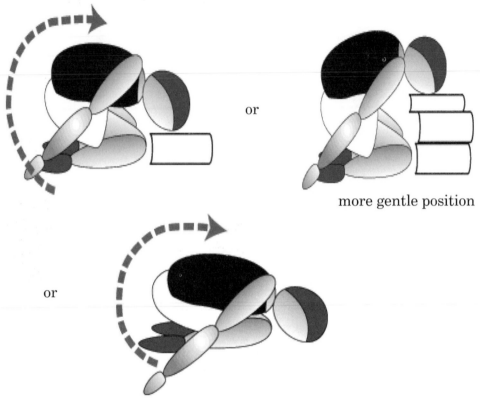

or

more gentle position

or

more advanced position

Exercise 15

16. Standing correctly and taking 12 complete breaths is a difficult exercise. It is not a waste of time, but an essential part of the back strengthening programme. Learn about your body as you stand still, be aware of the effect of the breath on your body, listen to your mind. Be aware as you work with these exercises, standing naturally, becoming more relaxed, feeling balance between both sides of the body. Imagine you are hanging from a ceiling. Gently lift the sternum diagonally upwards, not too much. Relax the arms against the body. Breathe and be aware.

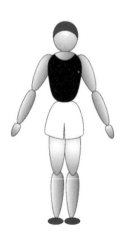

Exercise 16

17. Standing correctly, legs comfortably apart. As you inhale, bring the arms forward and above the head, forming a gentle U shape with the arms. Relax the shoulders. Slowly lower the arms sideways as you exhale.

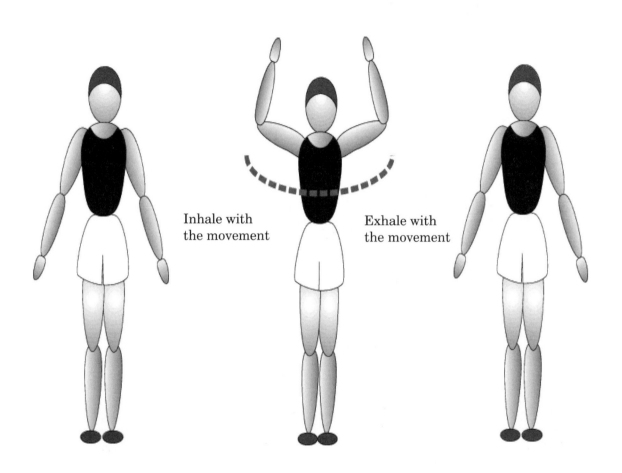

Inhale with
the movement

Exhale with
the movement

Exercise 17

18. The same as 17, but modifying to stretch more by bringing the hands together above the head and stretching up. Lower the arms sideways as you exhale.

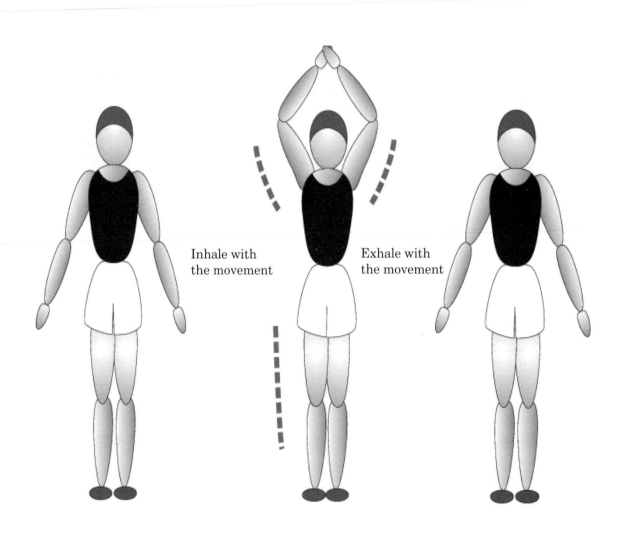

Inhale with the movement

Exhale with the movement

Exercise 18

19. This is the same as exercise 18, except that as you inhale and stretch the arms up, also rise on to the toes and stretch the legs. Try not to wobble, if you do, use a wall for support and use one hand to stretch upwards. Make sure you do the excerise in reverse, stretching up with the alternate hand.

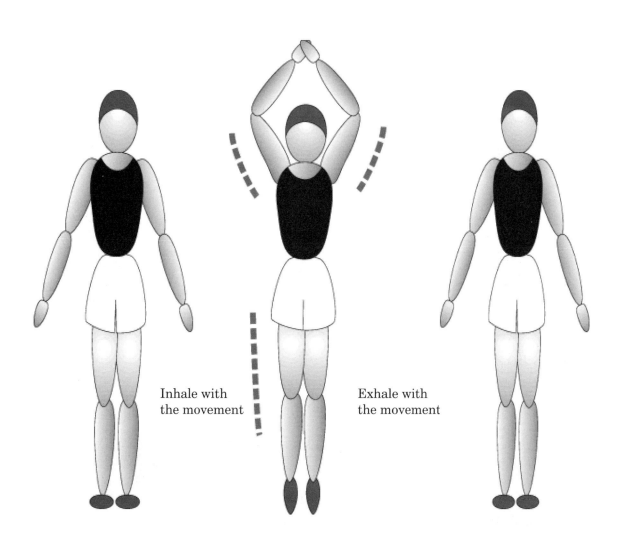

Inhale with
the movement

Exhale with
the movement

Exercise 19

20. Standing correctly, feet comfortably apart, inhale. Take the arms above the head, bend the knees a little. As you exhale, bend forward, taking the arms on to the back, folding the hands together on the back. Keeping the knees bent, begin to inhale, straightening the back, and the legs as you finish the movement. Lower the arms sideways as you exhale or, if you feel comfortable, go down again. Remember to keep the knees relaxed.

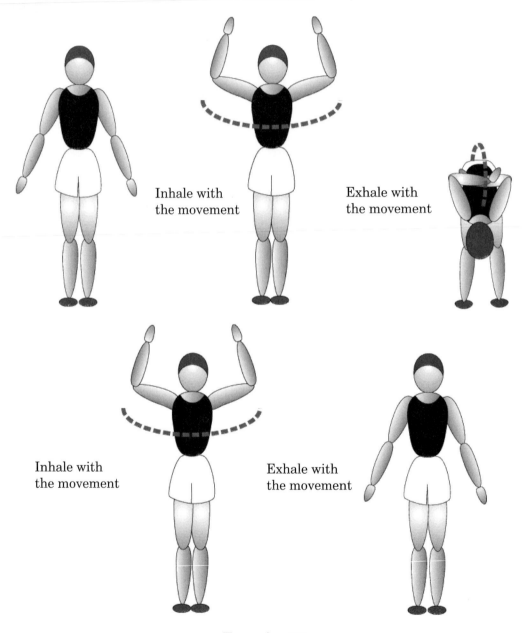

Inhale with the movement

Exhale with the movement

Inhale with the movement

Exhale with the movement

Exercise 20

This exercise can be modified. After sweeping the arms on to the back, gently uncurl the body as you inhale and return to the standing position.

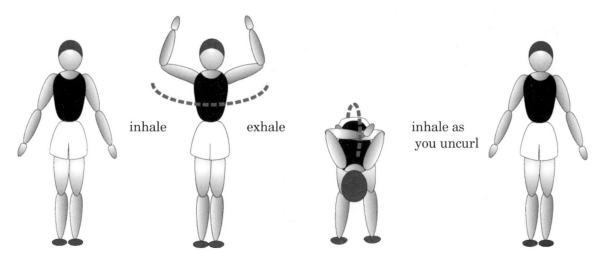

inhale   exhale   inhale as
                                you uncurl

Exercise 20a

21.   To gradually introduce a forward bending exercise into your back programme, use a chair to bend forward on to, and tuck one arm behind your back. As you inhale raise one arm above the head. Exhaling, bending the knees slightly, bend forward on to the chair. Inhaling, return to the standing position either by uncurling or stretching the body to return to a straight position.

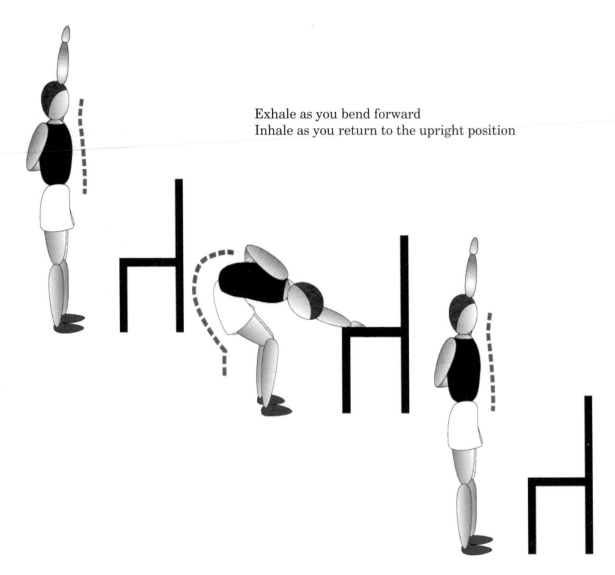

Exhale as you bend forward
Inhale as you return to the upright position

Exercise 21

Modify the exercise as you become stronger by not using the chair, and then with both arms together. It is very important to keep the knees bent when going into the forward bend, or out of it (see Exercise 21a).

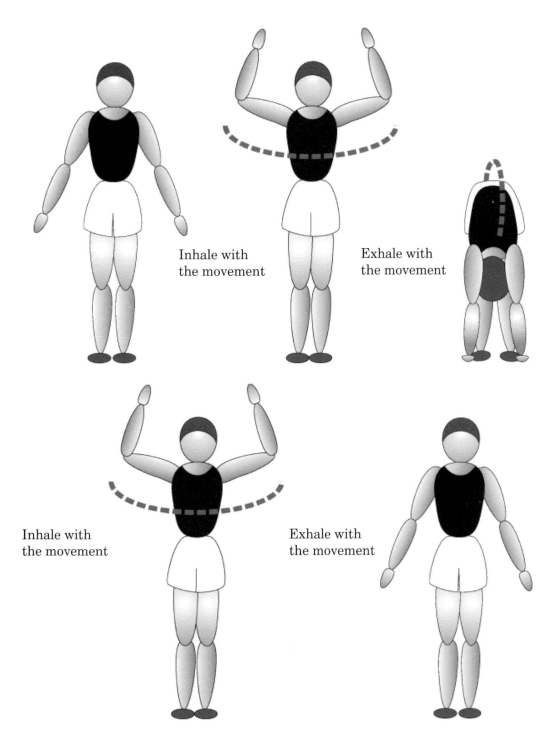

Inhale with
the movement

Exhale with
the movement

Inhale with
the movement

Exhale with
the movement

Exercise 21a

22. Take a pace forwards but do not overstretch. Place the arms behind you, resting on the waist area, keep the shoulders relaxed. Inhale, stretch up, lifting the body out of the pelvis area. Keep the legs light but firm and straight. Exhale slowly as you bend forward over one leg. Feel the stretch in the hamstrings. Inhale as you return to the straight position. This exercise is very important in your programme and must be approached with care and awareness.

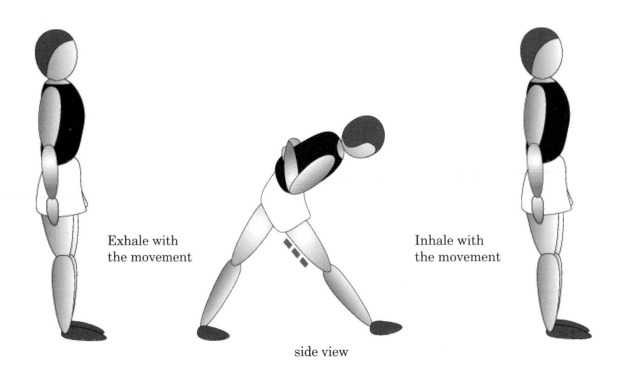

Exhale with
the movement

side view

Inhale with
the movement

Exercise 22

Note the foot position for this exercise

Feet face forwards one pace apart

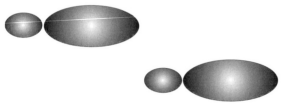

Front

As you gradually become more flexible, imagine you are pulling the bottom diagonally away from you. This increases the stretch on the hamstrings. Repeat on the other side. Do not feel work in any part of it the back leg. If you do, take a narrower pace and put a small paperback underneath the back heel.

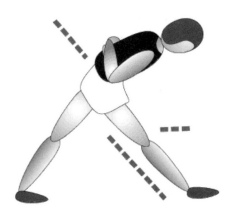

23. Take a pace sideways, put the feet into the correct position (see right). Inhale and stretch the body upwards. As you exhale, lower the body over the leg with the foot to the side. Allow the arm to stretch down the leg (left arm down left leg and vice versa). Allow the right arm to relax along the body. Keep the neck relaxed. Inhale, returning up to the straight position. Repeat with the other side. Modify the posture as you get stronger by keeping both arms straight.

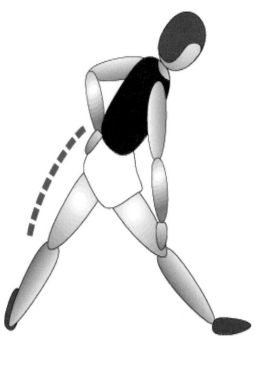

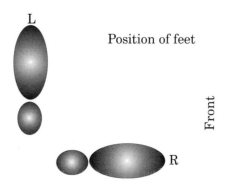

L

Position of feet

Front

R

Side view

Exercise 23

24. Keep the neck relaxed and allow the head to twist so that you look upwards when you are in the posture. Repeat with the other side.

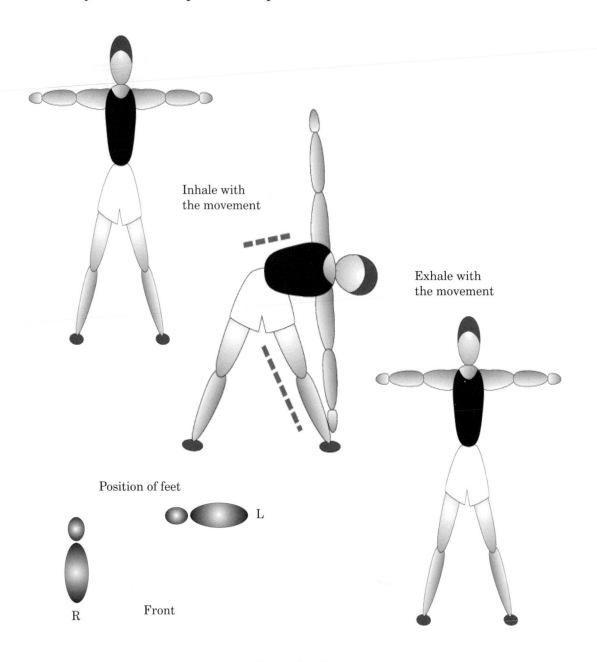

Inhale with
the movement

Exhale with
the movement

Position of feet

L

R   Front

Exercise 24

25. Standing with the feet apart, turn right foot to the right as shown. Bend the right knee over the right foot and slowly lower the body down over the bent knee. Bend the body down as you exhale and rise to the straight position as you inhale.

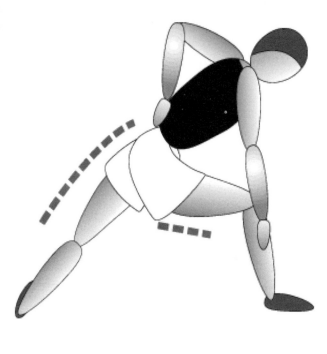

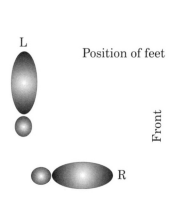

L

Position of feet

Front

R

Exercise 25

Modify the exercise by using straight arms (see Exercise 25a). Keep the neck relaxed and turned. Do not allow the knee to move past the right angle of the foot and leg. Repeat with the other side.

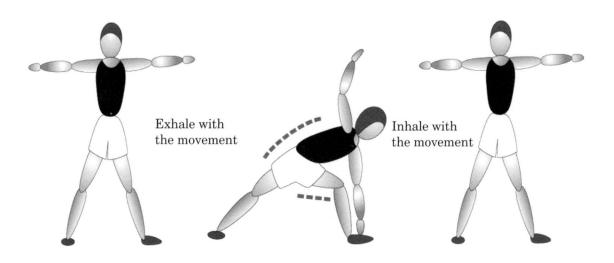

Exhale with the movement

Inhale with the movement

Exercise 25a

26. Stand with right leg forward, back leg straight. Bend the right knee over the right foot. Hold the hands together and draw them down towards the bottom. Stay in this position as you inhale deeply. This will tighten muscles under the lumbar area. Repeat with the other leg.

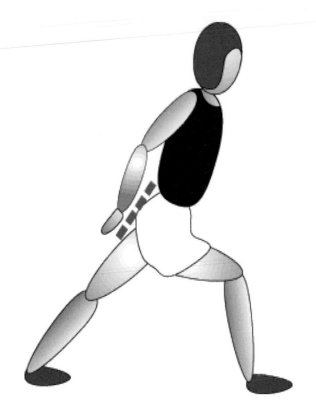

Inhale as the chest
draws forward.
Exhale and relax

Feet face forwards one pace apart

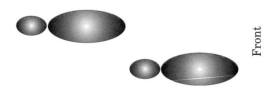

Front

Exercise 26

27. Stand with feet comfortably apart, relax the shoulders, inhale. Raise the arms above the head. Exhaling, lower the arms as you bend the knees allowing the body to go into a squat. Imagine you are sitting on a bar stool. Inhale, return to standing position with arms raised. Exhale, lower arms. Repeat. If you feel any work in the calf or ankle area, put a paperback book or two under the heels to support them when you squat down.

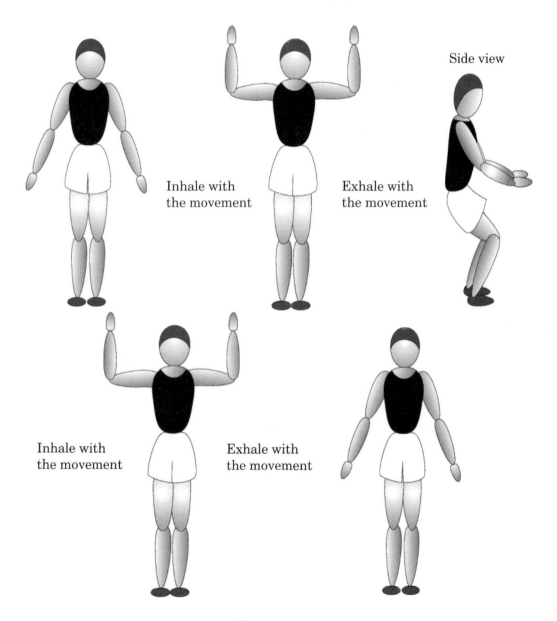

Side view

Inhale with
the movement

Exhale with
the movement

Inhale with
the movement

Exhale with
the movement

Exercise 27

28. Twisting movements can be made progressively harder as you develop strength and suppleness. It is, as always, important to work with the breathing. Stand with the legs comfortably apart and slowly twist as you exhale, allowing the body to relax and swing into the exercise.

To modify the exercise and make it harder, you need to cross the legs. This will keep the work in the back to a greater degree. Cross the left leg over the right leg and twist to the right as you exhale.

To modify this exercise to increase the difficulty cross the right leg over the left leg and twist to the right as you exhale. Remember, in both instances, to change the position of the feet before you twist the other way. If balance is a problem, hold on to a wall or a chair.

Therefore:

R/L twist to R = harder

L/R twist to R = easier.

Twist at the waist   R/L twist R   L/R twist R

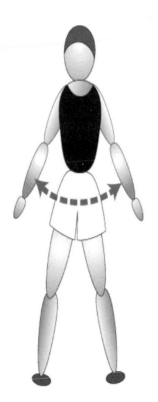 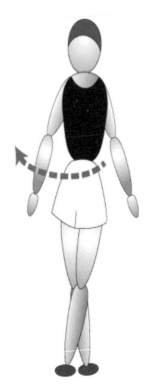 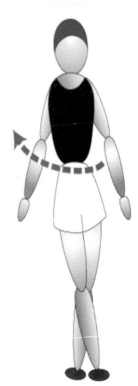

Modify

Exercise 28

29. Stand with your legs apart, feet facing forwards. Inhale, raise the arms above your head, stretching the backs of your legs and the spine. Exhaling, lower the body towards the floor slowly, stretching the hamstrings as you bend down. Uncurl the body as you return to the upright position also as you inhale. It is very important to feel the hamstrings work as you go down and remember to uncurlas you come upwards.

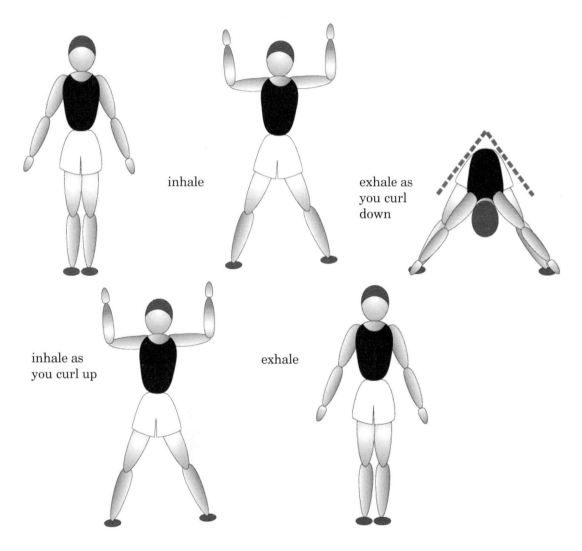

inhale

exhale as
you curl
down

inhale as
you curl up

exhale

Exercise 29

To modify this, use a chair to lower the body on to when you curl down (see *Figure 2.14*) and then as you gradually become stronger and more supple you will be able to curl down as in Exercise 29.

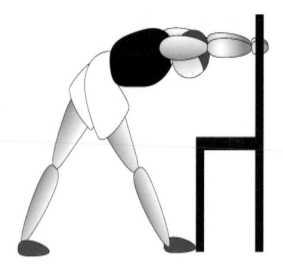

Figure 2.14

30. Lying on the stomach, relax the arms behind you on the floor and relax the legs. As you inhale, slowly stretch the neck and begin to lift the head and shoulders off the floor. You should feel the work in the abdominal area. Exhaling, lower the head and shoulders back to the floor. This exercise is often described in a misleading way. It is important that you do not allow the navel off the floor.

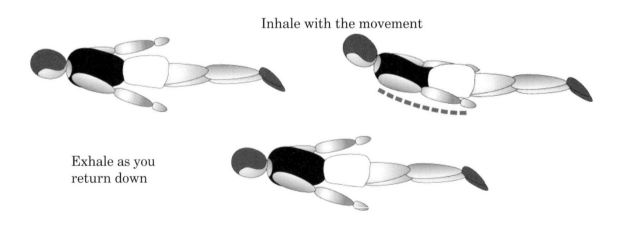

Inhale with the movement

Exhale as you return down

Exercise 30

You may modify this exercise by using the arms to help lift the body (see *Figure 2.15*). But remember, do not lift very high. Less work means more strength and flexibility.

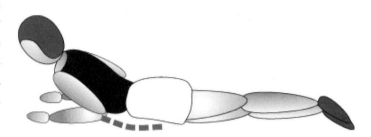

Figure 2.15

31. Lying on the side, with the head resting on an outstretched arm, support the body with the other arm. Inhale, lift the leg between 6" and 12". Exhale, lower the leg.

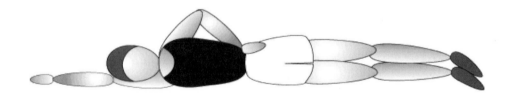

Inhale as you raise the leg

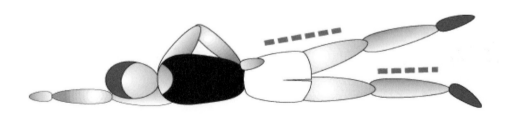

Exhale as you lower the leg
Repeat with the other leg

Exercise 31

32. As you inhale pull yourself up very straight. Bend the knee sideways and put the foot on the leg, just below the knee. Stay for one complete breath and lower the leg as you exhale. If needed place one hand one a wall to balance yourself. Repeat with the other leg.

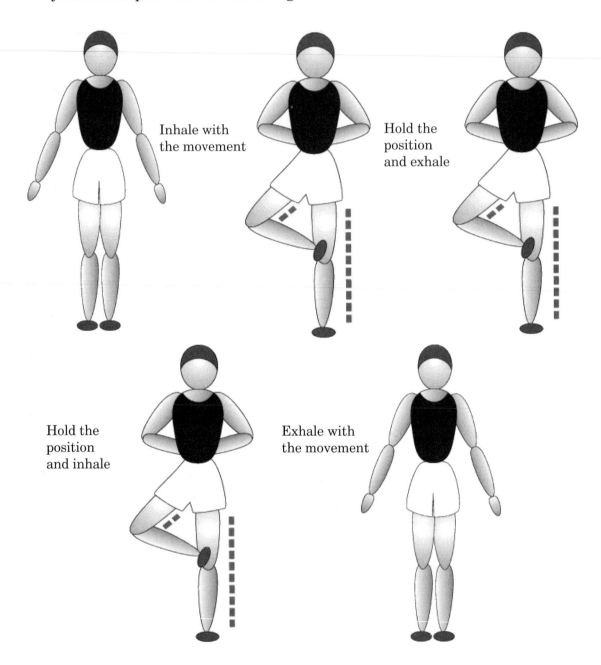

Inhale with the movement

Hold the position and exhale

Hold the position and inhale

Exhale with the movement

Exercise 32

33. Stand next to a wall. Bend the knee, grasp the ankle and raise it up to the buttock area to feel a stretch in your thigh. Repeat with the other leg.

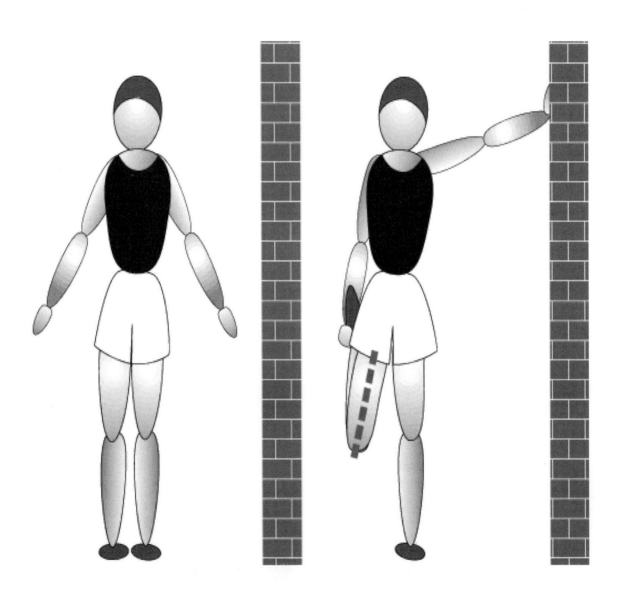

Exercise 33

34. Raise arms above the head and slowly lean forwards, using the wall for support. Extend one leg behind you and lift from the ground. Repeat with the other leg.

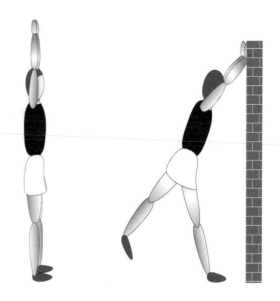

Exercise 34

35. Adominal curl. Lie on the back with the knees bent placing the hands either side of the head (see figure A). Alternatively relax the hands on to the thighs (see figure B). Draw the abdominals up towards the ribs. Feel as if the spine is touching the floor. Exhale as you lift head and shoulders approximately 6 inches at most from the floor. Inhale as you lower back to the floor.

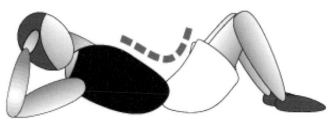

Figure A

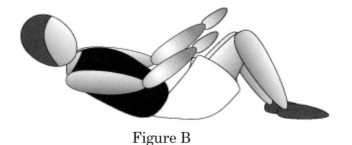

Figure B

Exercise 35

Sometimes it is beneficial to link the exercises in a sequence (*Figure 2.16*). Kneeling, inhale and stretch the arms forwards above the head. Exhale as you bend forwards and sweep the arms over and behind the head, relaxing them on the back. Inhale as you return to a kneeling position. Exhaling, lower the hands on to the floor. Inhaling, allow the waist to lower towards the floor. Exhaling, lower the body on to the legs, arms behind you. Inhaling, sit up. Repeat as many times as you need to. You may modify it by staying in an exercise for several breaths or repeating one that you enjoy.

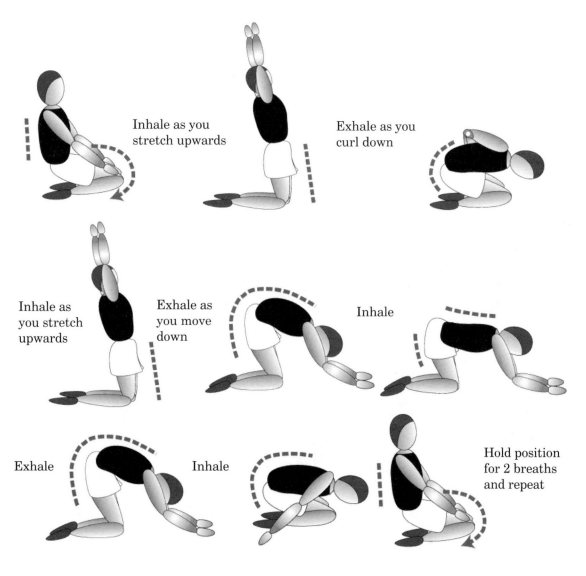

Figure 2.16

Beginning the exercise programme

These courses are important as they introduce the body to exercise and give the back an initial strength which will enable you to use the exercise programmes. Refer back to the exercise section if you are in doubt over any of these exercises.

Course 1

1.

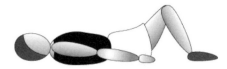

Remain in this position and take 6 breaths

2.

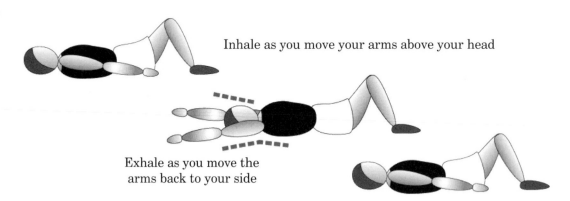

Inhale as you move your arms above your head

Exhale as you move the arms back to your side

3.

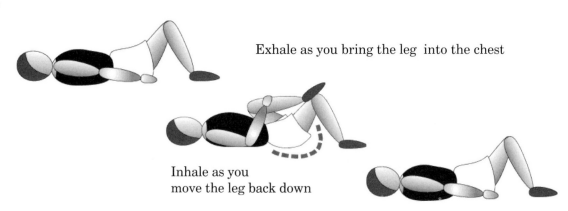

Exhale as you bring the leg into the chest

Inhale as you move the leg back down

4.

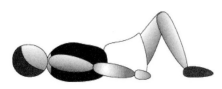

Exhale as you bring the leg into the chest

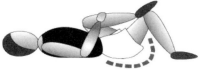

Inhale as you extend the leg

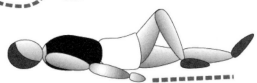

5.

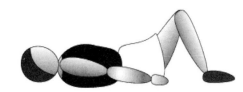

Inhale as you lift the bottom from the floor

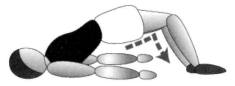

Exhale as you lower back to the floor

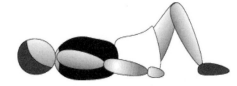

6.

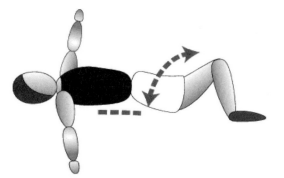

Lying twist
Repeat up to 6 times
each side

7.

Remain in the
position and take
6 breaths

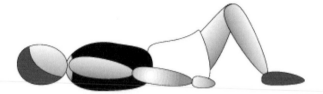

8.

Pelvis tilt

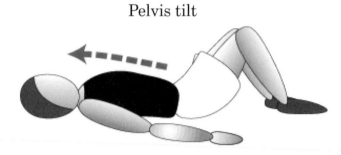

Ease the lower back into the floor and allow the pelvis to tilt upward —
pause and release. Repeat up to 6 times

9.

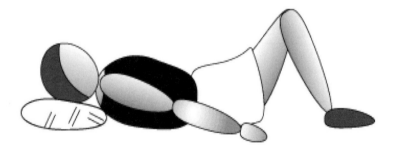

Remain in the position and take 12 breaths
Really concentrate releasing unnecessary tension
from the body which each breath.

When you are completely at ease with this course start on the next stage. Do not
hurry; move slowly and remember to use the breath. Repeat each exercise as many
times as you feel you safely can. Have patience.

Course 2

This course is a little harder and will continue to develop back strength. Repeat these exercises every day until you feel strong enough to progress to the next course in your *Back to Strength* programme.

1.

Remain in this position and take 12 breaths. Focus on lengthening your breaths and making each one deeper

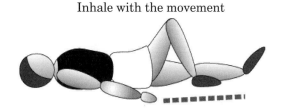

2.

Inhale with the movement

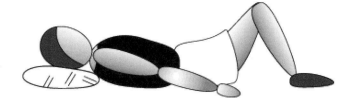

Exhale with the movement

Hold the leg in the position as you inhale point toes towards your face

Exhale with the movement

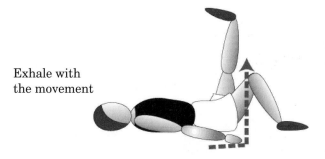

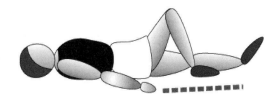

3.

Exhale as you raise your leg

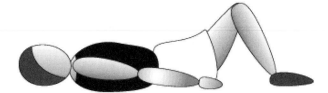

Stay in this position
as you inhale

Exhale as you lower your leg
Repeat 3 times with each leg

4.   Slowly open and close the legs 2–4 times

Inhale as you open the legs

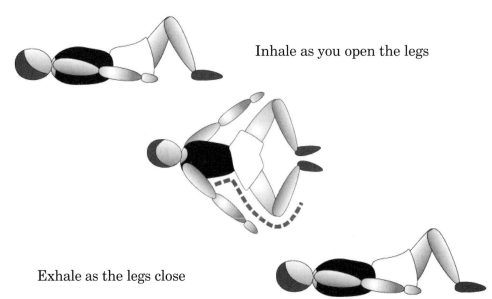

Exhale as the legs close

5.

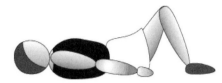

Inhale as you lift the bottom from the floor

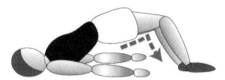

Exhale as you lower back to the floor

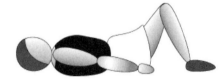

6.

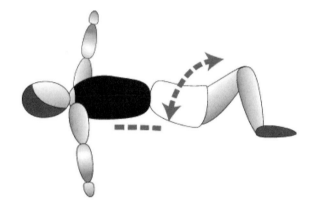

Lying twist

Repeat up to 6 times on each side

7.

8.

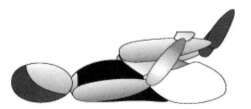

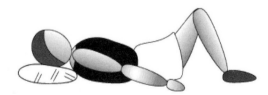

Ease the knees in towards the chest. Remain in this position and take 6 breaths

Remain in the position and take 12 breaths

Course 3

1.

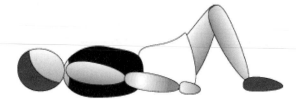

Remain in this position and take 6 breaths

2.

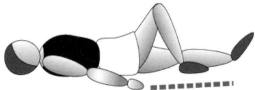

Exhale as you raise the leg

Hold the leg in the upright position and inhale. As you take the breath pull the toes towards the face. Reppeat 3–4 times with each leg

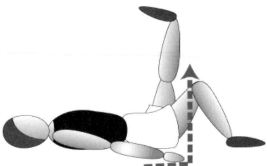

3.

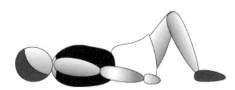

Inhale as you lift your bottom from the floor

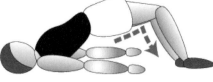

Exhale as you lower back to the floor

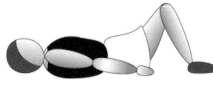

Repeat 3–6 times

4.

A

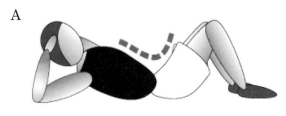

Lie on the back with the knees
bent placing the hands either at the
side of the head (see figure A) or
relaxed upon the thighs
(see figure B). Exhale as you lift
head and shoulders approximately
6inches at most from the floor.
Inhale as your lower the head to
back to the floor.
Repeat between 2–6 times.

B

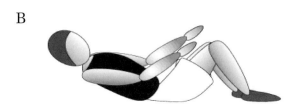

5.

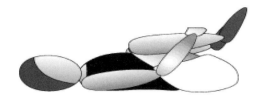

Hold this position and take 6 breaths

6.

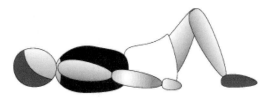

Remain in this position and
take 6 breaths

Proceed to Course 4 only when you are strong enough to do so.

Course 4

Use this programme until you can work with the exercises easily. As this is a more difficult course you should build up the the repetitions. Begin by repeating the movements 2–3 times and then increase the repetitions as you become stronger and more flexible. As usual, work with the breath and slowly. If you feel any pain stop.

1.

Stand and take
6 breaths

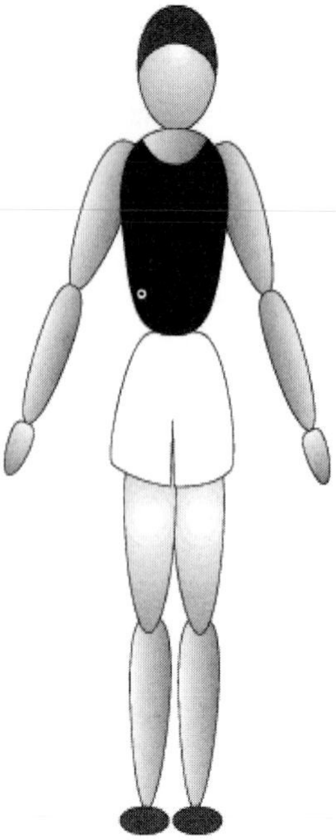

2.

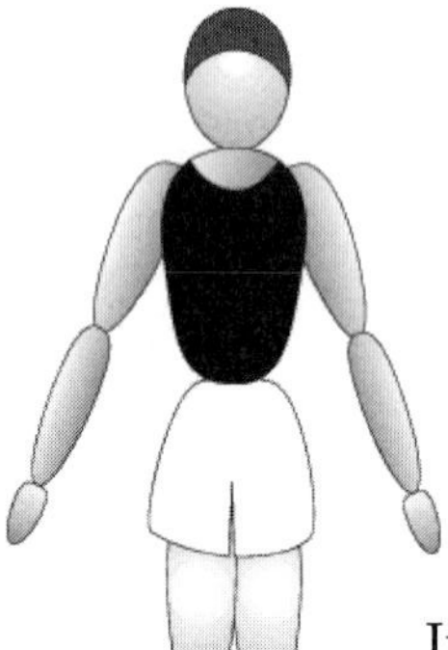

Inhale as you
sweep your arms
above your head

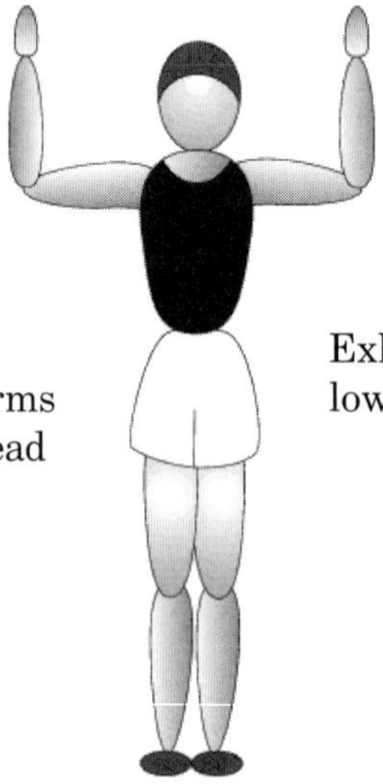

Exhale as you
lower the arms

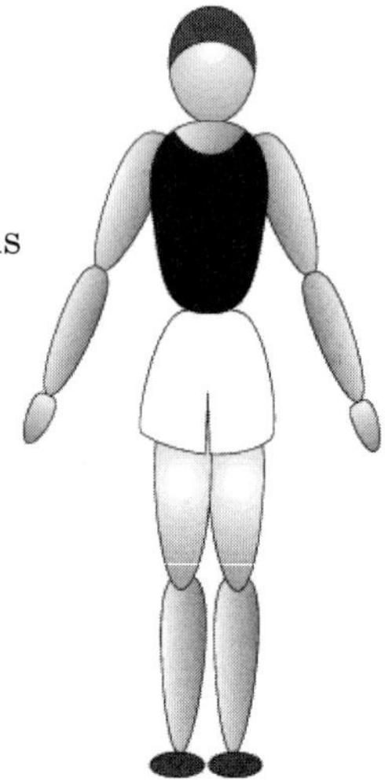

Repeat 6 times

3.

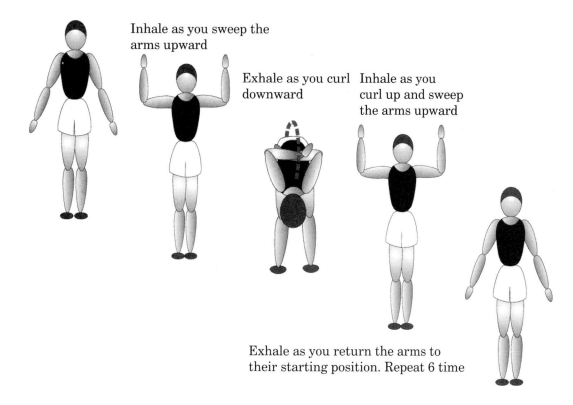

Inhale as you sweep the arms upward

Exhale as you curl downward

Inhale as you curl up and sweep the arms upward

Exhale as you return the arms to their starting position. Repeat 6 time

4.

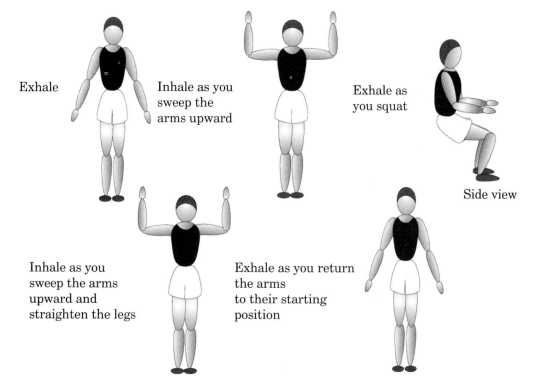

Exhale

Inhale as you sweep the arms upward

Exhale as you squat

Side view

Inhale as you sweep the arms upward and straighten the legs

Exhale as you return the arms to their starting position

5.

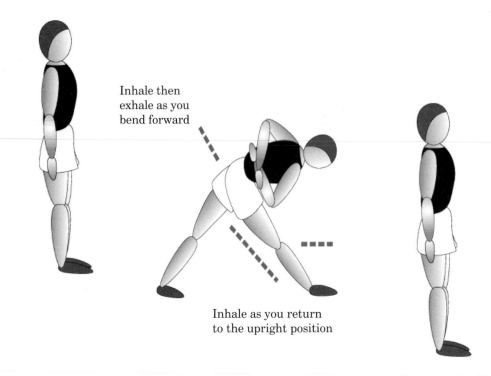

Inhale then
exhale as you
bend forward

Inhale as you return
to the upright position

6.

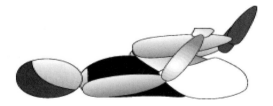

Exhale as you bring the legs into
the chest. Remain in this position
this position and take 6 breaths

7.

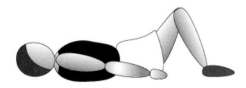

Inhale as you lift the bottom from
the floor

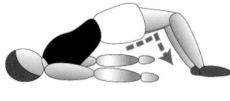

Exhale as you lower
the bottom back
to the floor.

Repeat 6 times

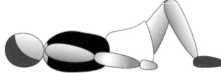

8.

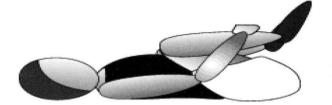

Exhale as you bring the legs
into the chest. Remain in this
position and take 6 breaths

9.

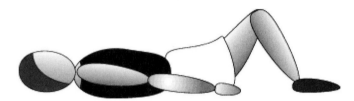

Remain in this position
and take 12 breaths

When beginning this course it is best to use between 2–3 repetitions and to build up
to the prescribed amount of repetitions. As usual work slowly and with the breath.
Stop if you feel any pain. Use this programme until you can work with the exercises
easily.

Section 3

Exercise programmes

This section includes:

- Exercises for energy
- Exercises for legs
- Exercises for suppleness
- Exercises for the abdomen
- Exercises for pelvic stability
- Exercises for the neck and shoulders
- Exercises for relaxation
- Exercises to relieve tension caused by remaining in one position too long
- Eight-day maintenance plans
- Relaxation techniques
- Final advice.

Exercise programmes for specific problems

The following exercise programmes are each designed to target a specific problem area. They include programmes for energy, the legs, the abdomen, the pelvis and the neck and shoulders. Each programme will allow you to focus on that problem area in order to alleviate the pain and to strengthen that area. Initially it may prove useful to refer back to the description of each exercise so that you make sure you are performing each exercise correctly.

Exercises for energy

1.

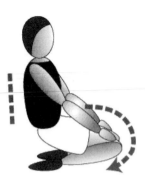

Take 6–12 breaths. Concentrate on inhalation. Try to lengthen and deepen each breath

2.

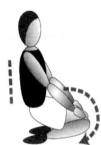

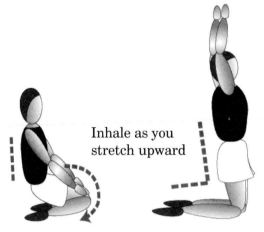

Inhale as you stretch upward

Exhale as you move back down

Repeat 6 times

3.

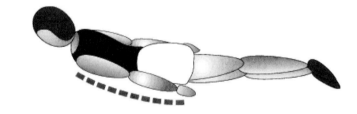

Inhale as you lift up. Repeat 6 times

4.

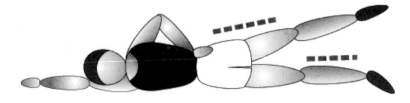

Inhale as you raise the leg. Lift leg 6 times
Repeat with the other leg

5.

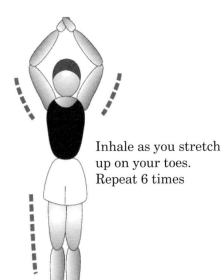

Inhale as you stretch up on your toes. Repeat 6 times

6. Take a step forward. Inhale with the movement

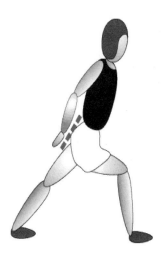

Repeat 3–6 times with each leg

7.

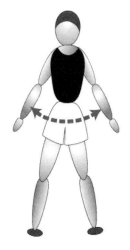

Twist 6 times each side

8.

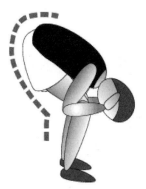

Exhale as you bend forward. Repeat 6 times

9.

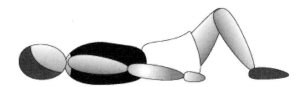

Take 12 breaths. Concentrate on inhalation and your affirmation

Exercises for the legs

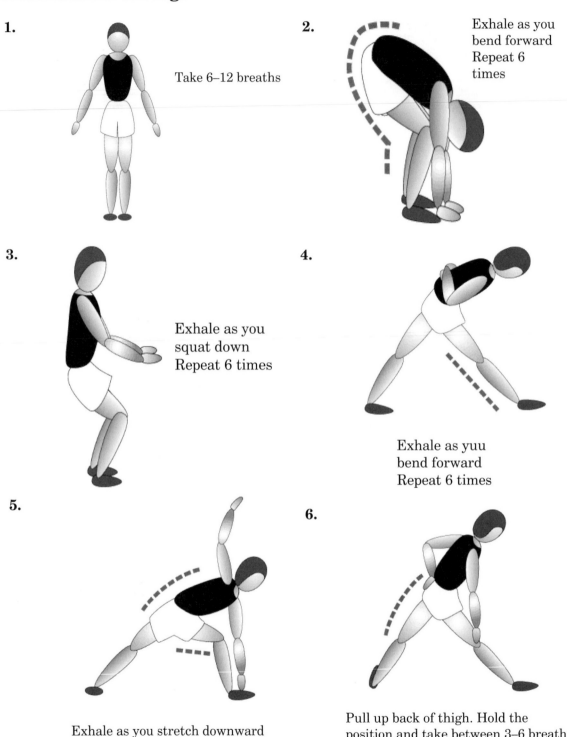

1.

Take 6–12 breaths

2.

Exhale as you
bend forward
Repeat 6
times

3.

Exhale as you
squat down
Repeat 6 times

4.

Exhale as yuu
bend forward
Repeat 6 times

5.

Exhale as you stretch downward
Repeat 6 times on each side

6.

Pull up back of thigh. Hold the
position and take between 3–6 breaths

7.

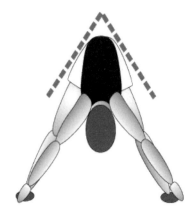

Exhale as you bend forward
Remain in the position for
3–6 breaths Uncurl to come up

8.

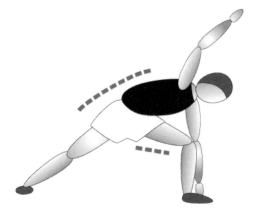

Exhale with movement
Repeat 3–6 times on each leg

9.

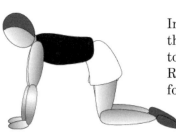

Inhale as you pull
the pelvis up
toward the ceiling.
Remain in this position
for 3–6 breaths

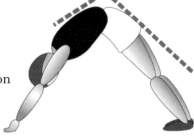

10.

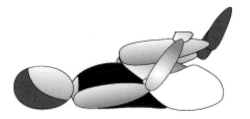

Bring your knees in to the chest.
Remain in the position and
take 6 breaths.

11.

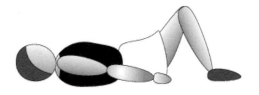

Stay in this position
take 12 breaths

Exercises for suppleness

If kneeling is a problem due to knees that are not supple, or are painful, or if you have varicose veins, use a pillow under your knees and/or between the bottom and the heels.

1.

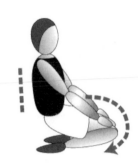

Hold the position for 6 breaths

2.

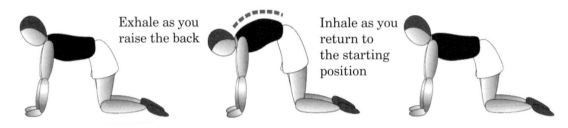

Exhale as you raise the back

Inhale as you return to the starting position

Repeat at least 6 times

3.

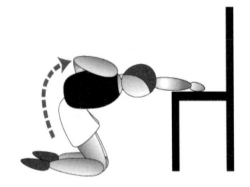

You can remove the chair to increase the difficulty and thereby increase your suppleness
Repeat 3 times with each arm

4.

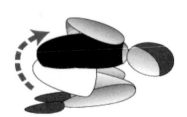

Repeat 6 times

5.

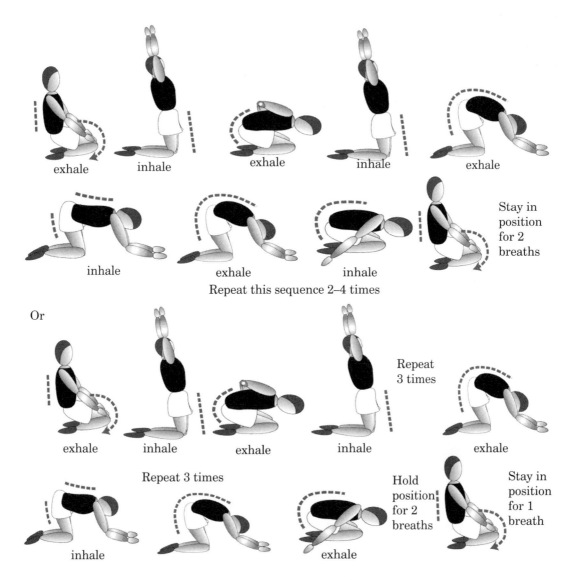

exhale inhale exhale inhale exhale

inhale exhale inhale Stay in position for 2 breaths

Repeat this sequence 2–4 times

Or

exhale inhale exhale inhale Repeat 3 times exhale

Repeat 3 times

inhale exhale Hold position for 2 breaths Stay in position for 1 breath

6.

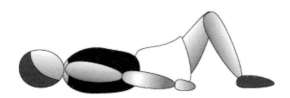

Take 12 breaths

Exercises for the abdomen

Exercises for the abdomen are very important. However, you must work with care and great awareness and with the breath. Vulnerable areas, such as the neck and lower back must be protected by being aware of what you are doing. Repeat the exercises as many times as you feel you can without discomfort. Stop when your body tells you 'enough'. Build up the number of repetitions gradually. Being overweight is detrimental to abdominal muscles. Correct posture will also help to strengthen the abdominals.

1.

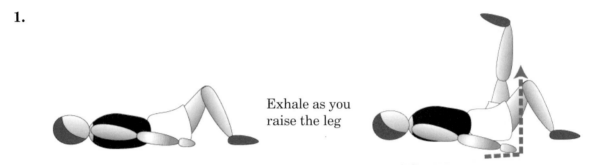

Exhale as you raise the leg

Move the leg on the exhalation. Repeat 3–6 times

2.

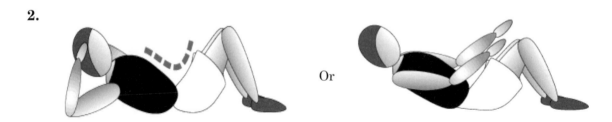

Or

Remember to visualise where the work is going. Concentrate upon this area. Think about the abdominal muscles working, tightening. Do not use the neck or shoulders to lift up. Repeat as necessary

3.

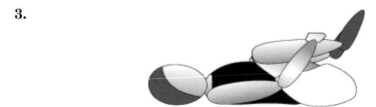

Exhale as you bring your knees in to your chest.
Remain in this position and take 6 breaths

4.

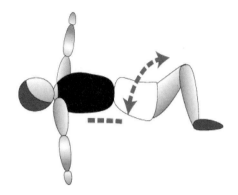

Twist to each side

To modify this exercise to make it more difficult place the foot on the opposite knee and take the bent knee across the body as you exhale. Return to the centre when you inhale. Change position of the foot to work the other side.

5.

Exhale as you raise one leg and gently circle the extended foot lengthways.
Repeat using the other leg as necessary.

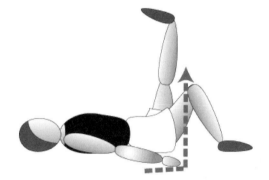

6.

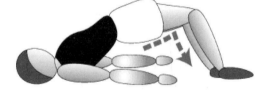

7.

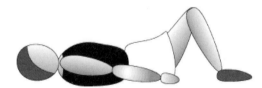

Exhale with the movement.
Repeat 6 times

Take 12 breaths

Exercises for pelvic stability

Balance exercises are extremely important when developing pelvic stability as it is essential to work the weak side of the body independently from the strong side. However, these exercises must be approached with caution.This type of exercise may cause difficulty: if you wobble you may actually damage your back further. Therefore unless you are certain you can stand balanced on one leg without a single wobble use a chair for support. Do not hang on to the chair but just use your hand on it or alternatively rest you hand on a wall. To aid balance fix your gaze and hold it on a point that is level with your natural eye level. Concentrate on the exhalation and breath slowly.

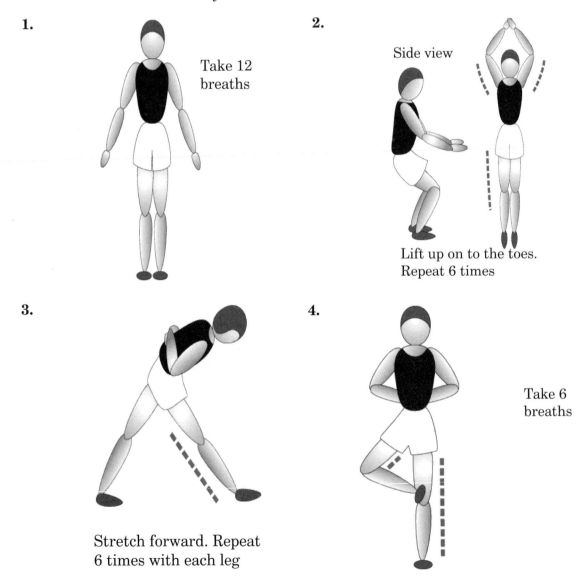

1.

Take 12 breaths

2.

Side view

Lift up on to the toes. Repeat 6 times

3.

Stretch forward. Repeat 6 times with each leg

4.

Take 6 breaths

5.

Take 12
breaths

6.

Side view

Lift up on to the toes.
Repeat 6 times

7.

Stretch forward. Repeat
6 times with each leg

8.

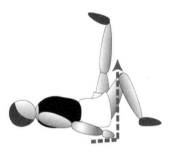

Ease the leg toward the chest
3–6 times with each leg.

9.

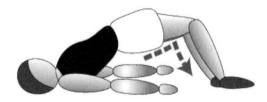

Repeat 6 times

10.

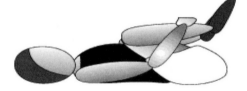

Exhale as you bring the
knees in to the chest.
Remain in the position and take
6 breaths.

11.

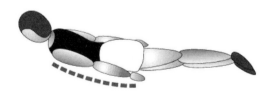

Repeat 6 times

12.

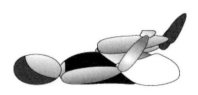

Exhale as bring the knees in to
the chest.
Hold the position and take 12 breaths

Exercises for the neck and shoulders

Neck and shoulder problems are often the result of tension in the trapezius muscles and of pelvic instability. Even if the pain is the result of injury, tension will retain the pain and result in lack of mobility in this area. Neck and pelvis, lower back pain and neck and shoulder problems must be identified and rectified together. One must try to obtain pelvic stability when trying to help the neck/shoulder area. Therefore it may prove helpful to work with the exercises for pelvic stability and the neck and shoulders together.

1.

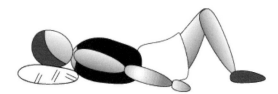

Take 12 breaths. Visualise the tight areas of your body relaxing.

2.

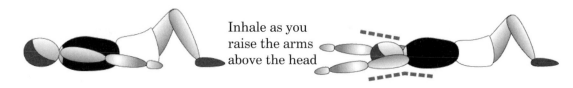

Inhale as you raise the arms above the head

Repeat 6 times

3.

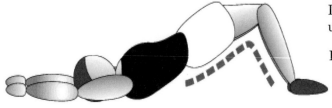

Inhale as you raise your body upward making a gentle U shape

Repeat 6 times

4.

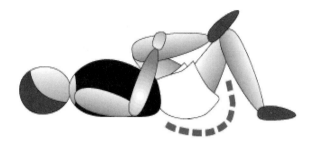

Gently lift the head forwards towards the knee.
Repeat 3 times with each leg

5.

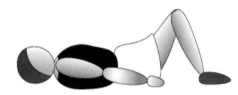

Take 12 breaths

6.

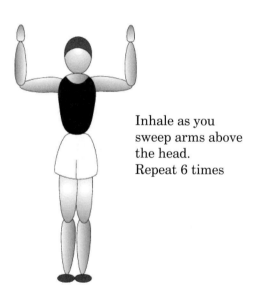

Inhale as you sweep arms above the head.
Repeat 6 times

7.

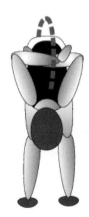

Exhale as you curl downward.
Uncurl to return to standing.
Repeat 6 times

8.

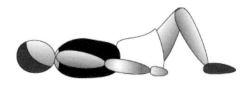

Take 12 breaths

Exercises for relaxation

1.

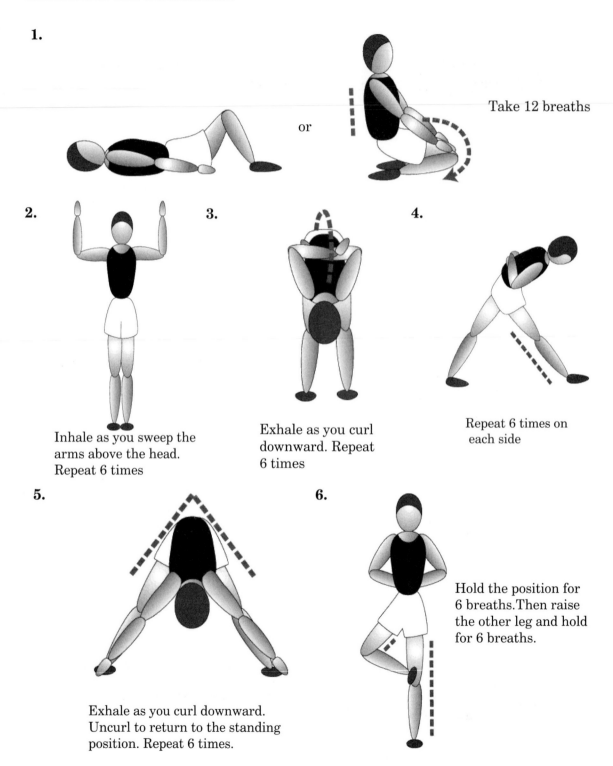

or

Take 12 breaths

2.

Inhale as you sweep the
arms above the head.
Repeat 6 times

3.

Exhale as you curl
downward. Repeat
6 times

4.

Repeat 6 times on
each side

5.

Exhale as you curl downward.
Uncurl to return to the standing
position. Repeat 6 times.

6.

Hold the position for
6 breaths. Then raise
the other leg and hold
for 6 breaths.

7.

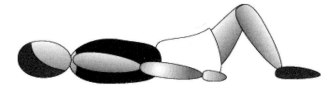

Take 12 breaths

8.

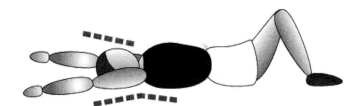

Inhale as the arms are
raised above the head.
Repeat 6 times

9.

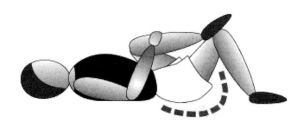

Repeat 6 times with each leg

10.

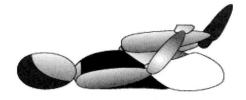

Exhale as you bring the knees
in to the chest.
Hold the position and take 6 breaths

11.

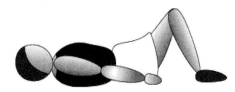

Take 12–24 breaths. Stretch gently to release.
Move slowly. It is essential to concentrate
on the exhalation during these exercises

Exercises to relieve tension in the spine caused by too much sitting in one position

1.

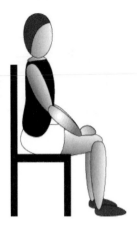

Take 12 breaths.
Concentrate on stretching the spine with each inhalation

2.

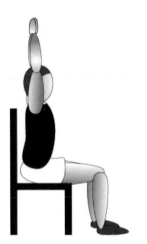

Inhale as you stretch the arms upward.
Repeat 6 times

3.

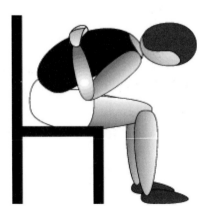

Exhale as you curl forward placing the arms behind your back. Inhale as you return to the upright position.
Repeat 6 times

4.

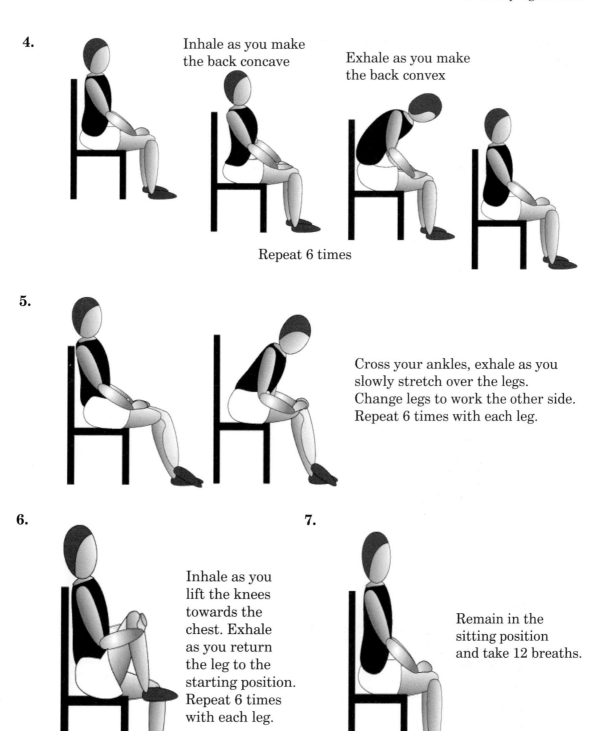

Inhale as you make
the back concave

Exhale as you make
the back convex

Repeat 6 times

5.

Cross your ankles, exhale as you
slowly stretch over the legs.
Change legs to work the other side.
Repeat 6 times with each leg.

6.

Inhale as you
lift the knees
towards the
chest. Exhale
as you return
the leg to the
starting position.
Repeat 6 times
with each leg.

7.

Remain in the
sitting position
and take 12 breaths.

Eight-day maintenance plan

This exercise programme is an eight-day sequence plan. This is in order to avoid your doing the same exercise on the same day every week and becoming bored. Apathy and boredom are a risk and you must remain aware and be fresh every time you work with your exercises. You may question the necessity of regular practise. However, if you think back to the discomfort of a bad back and the fact that doing these exercises regularly alleviates the pain then you will not neglect to perform these exercises regularly. Exercise or pain will return.

You must stretch slowly and work with the breath during every exercise. Remember your positive affirmation before you begin each day's new exercise plan. This will help you to achieve a positive mind-set.

It is important that you make the exercises part of your daily routine. One day missed is potentially a step on the slippery slope towards returning to having a back problem. It is as simple as *brush your teeth, wash your face, do your exercises.*

Remember to repeat each exercise as many times as you feel comfortable that day. There is no set number of repetions for each exercise. It depends on how you feel emotionally, mentally and physically, and these factors will vary from day to day. Adjust your practice accordingly. Re-read the exercise notes to familiarise yourself on how to work with the exercises correctly. Each day should take between 10 and 15 minutes depending on how you feel.

There are two eight-day maintenance exercise programmes. The first one is more gentle and contains easier exercises for when you feel stressed or tired or are recovering from an illness. The second eight-day plan is harder and should be used to maintain your strength and suppleness.

Exercise with awareness. Breathe correctly. Remember your affirmation. Always exercise within the limits of pain.

Eight-day maintenance plan — gentle

Day 1: repeat exercises 2–6 times each

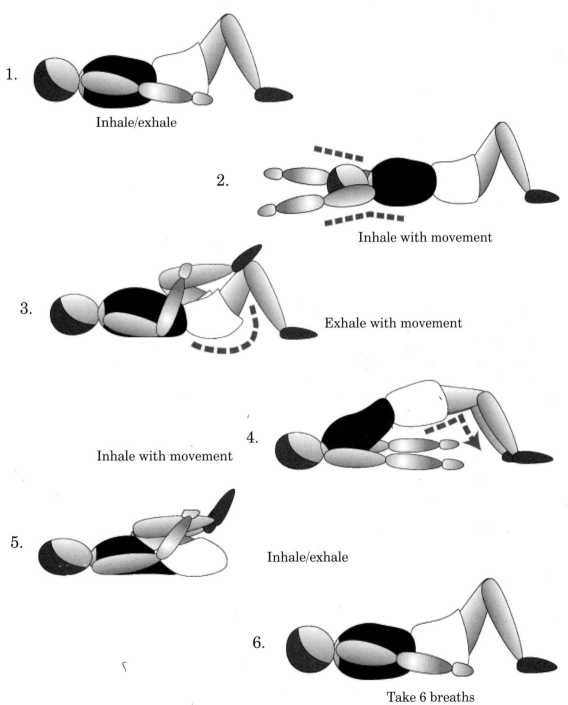

1. Inhale/exhale

2. Inhale with movement

3. Exhale with movement

4. Inhale with movement

5. Inhale/exhale

6. Take 6 breaths

Day 2: repeat exercises 2–6 times each

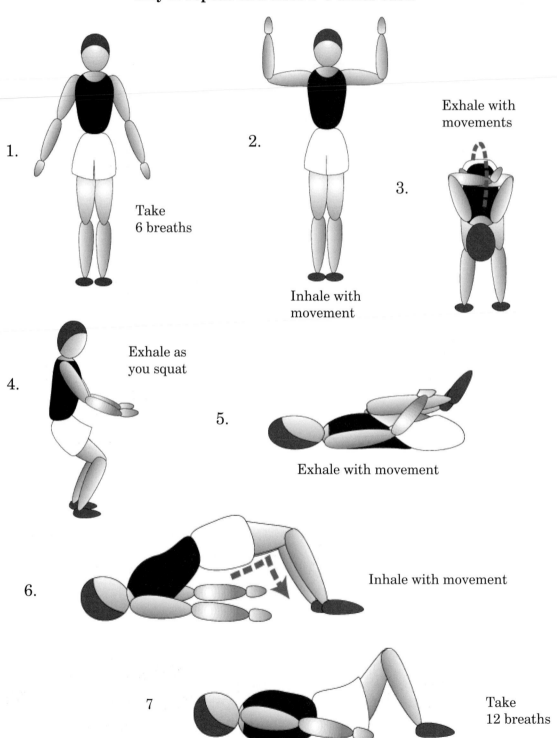

1.

Take
6 breaths

2.

Inhale with
movement

Exhale with
movements

3.

4.

Exhale as
you squat

5.

Exhale with movement

6.

Inhale with movement

7

Take
12 breaths

Day 3: repeat exercises 2–6 times each

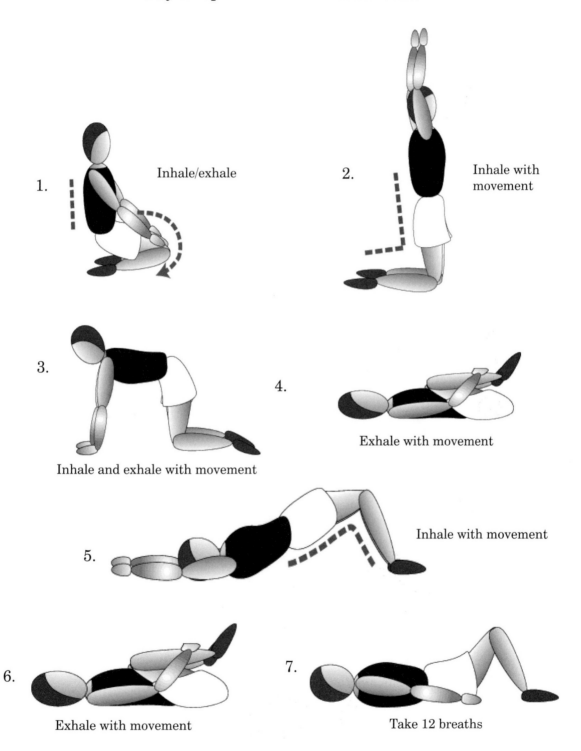

1. Inhale/exhale

2. Inhale with movement

3. Inhale and exhale with movement

4. Exhale with movement

5. Inhale with movement

6. Exhale with movement

7. Take 12 breaths

Day 4: repeat exercises 2–6 times each

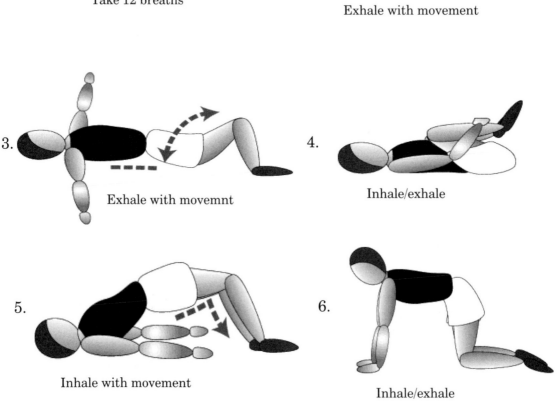

1. Take 12 breaths

2. Exhale with movement

3. Exhale with movemnt

4. Inhale/exhale

5. Inhale with movement

6. Inhale/exhale

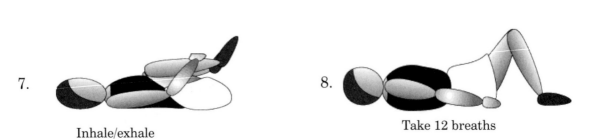

7. Inhale/exhale

8. Take 12 breaths

Day 5: repeat exercise 2–6 times each

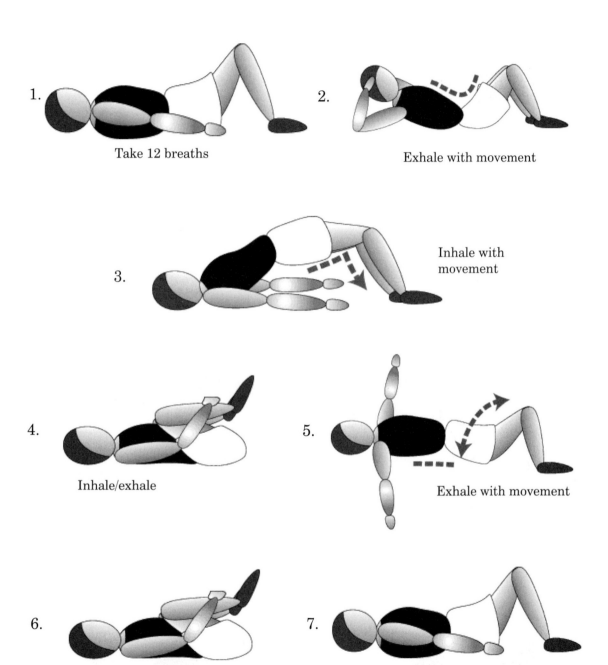

1. Take 12 breaths

2. Exhale with movement

3. Inhale with movement

4. Inhale/exhale

5. Exhale with movement

6. Inhale/exhale

7. Take 12 breaths

Day 6: repeat exercises 2–6 times each

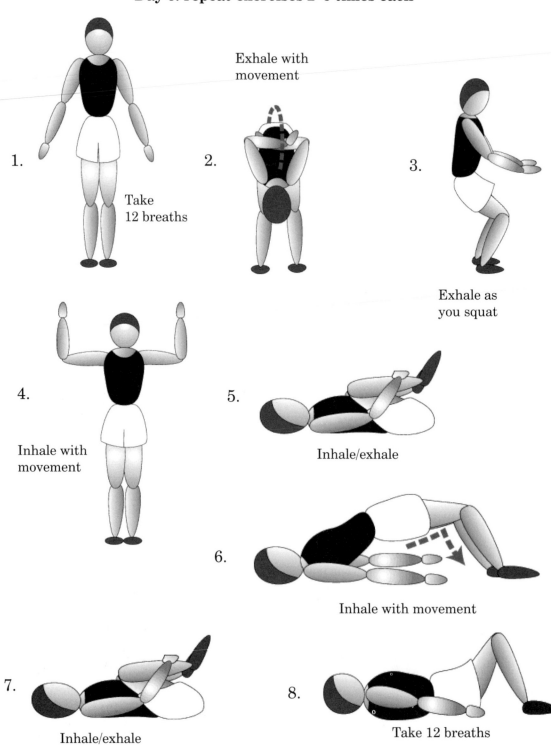

1.

Take
12 breaths

Exhale with
movement

2.

3.

Exhale as
you squat

4.

Inhale with
movement

5.

Inhale/exhale

6.

Inhale with movement

7.

Inhale/exhale

8.

Take 12 breaths

Day 7: repeat this sequence 2–6 times

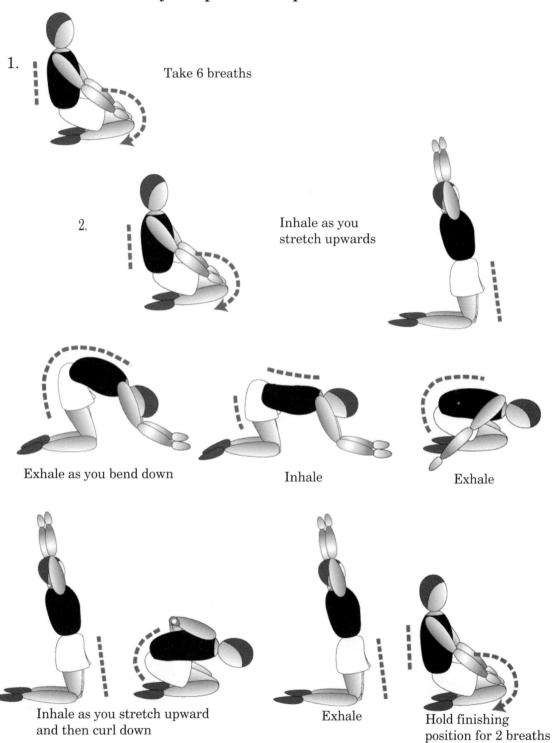

1. Take 6 breaths

2. Inhale as you stretch upwards

Exhale as you bend down

Inhale

Exhale

Inhale as you stretch upward and then curl down

Exhale

Hold finishing position for 2 breaths

Day 8: repeat exercises 2–6 times each

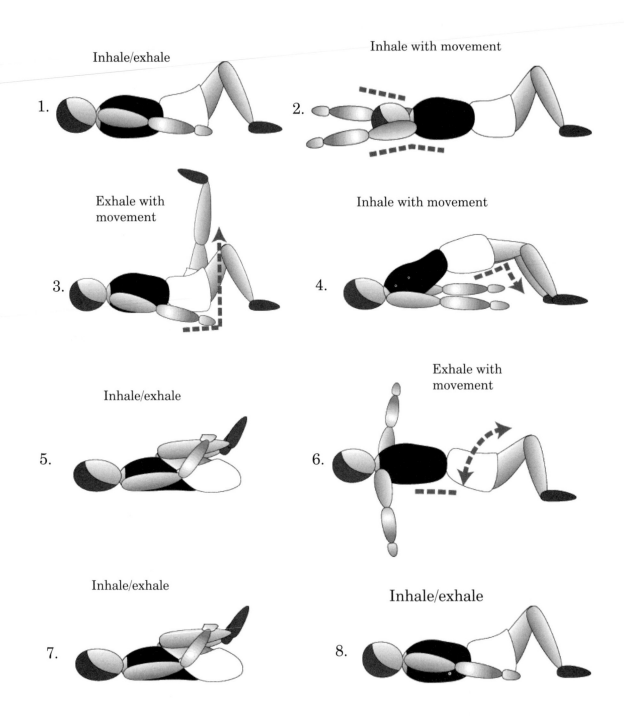

Inhale/exhale

1.

Inhale with movement

2.

Exhale with movement

3.

Inhale with movement

4.

Inhale/exhale

5.

Exhale with movement

6.

Inhale/exhale

7.

Inhale/exhale

8.

Eight-day maintenance plan – regular

Day 1: repeat exercises 2–6 times each

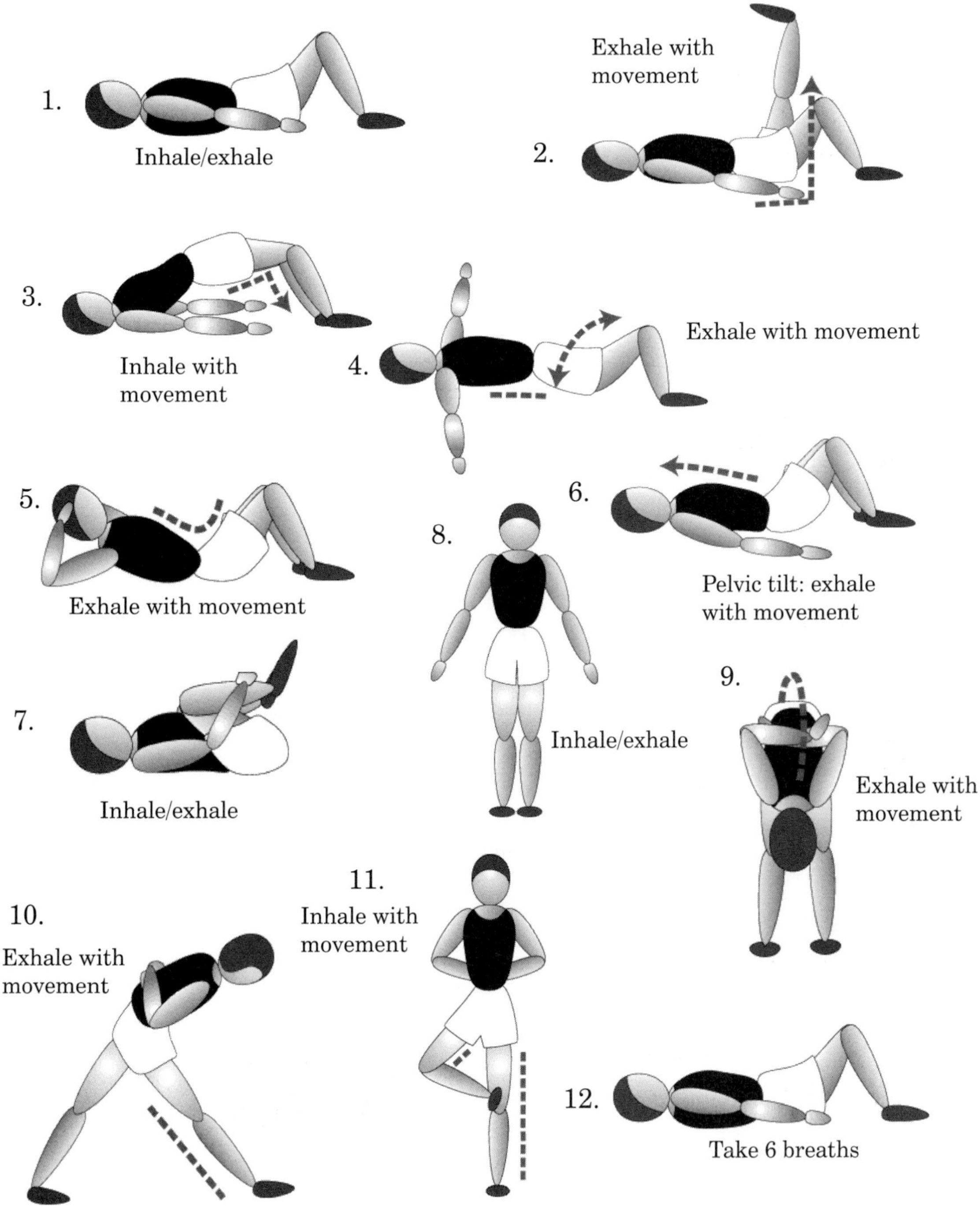

1. Inhale/exhale

2. Exhale with movement

3. Inhale with movement

4. Exhale with movement

5. Exhale with movement

6. Pelvic tilt: exhale with movement

7. Inhale/exhale

8. Inhale/exhale

9. Exhale with movement

10. Exhale with movement

11. Inhale with movement

12. Take 6 breaths

Day 2: repeat exercises 2–6 times each

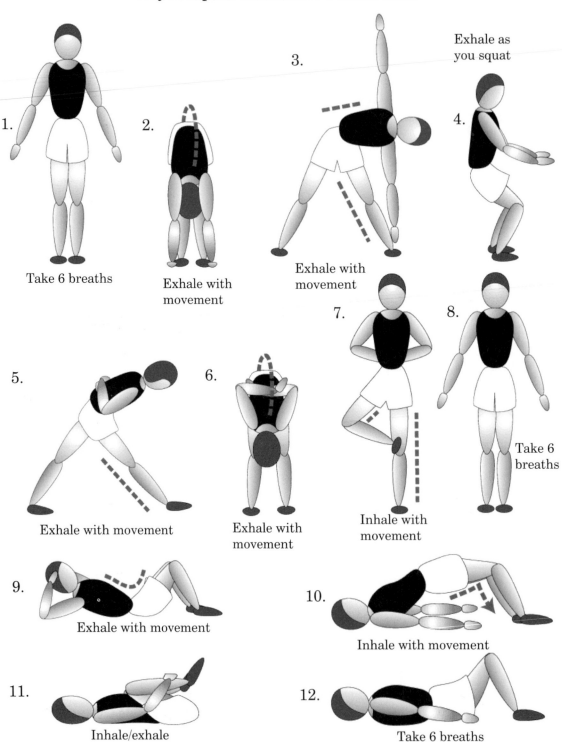

1. Take 6 breaths

2. Exhale with movement

3. Exhale with movement

4. Exhale as you squat

5. Exhale with movement

6. Exhale with movement

7. Inhale with movement

8. Take 6 breaths

9. Exhale with movement

10. Inhale with movement

11. Inhale/exhale

12. Take 6 breaths

Day 3: repeat exercises 2–6 times each

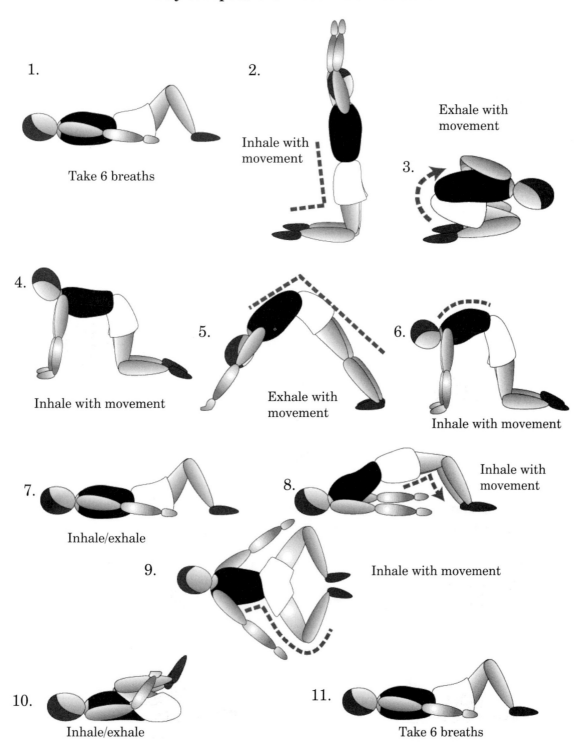

1.

Take 6 breaths

2.

Inhale with movement

Exhale with movement

3.

4.

Inhale with movement

5.

Exhale with movement

6.

Inhale with movement

7.

Inhale/exhale

8.

Inhale with movement

9.

Inhale with movement

10.

Inhale/exhale

11.

Take 6 breaths

Day 4: repeat exercises 2–6 times each

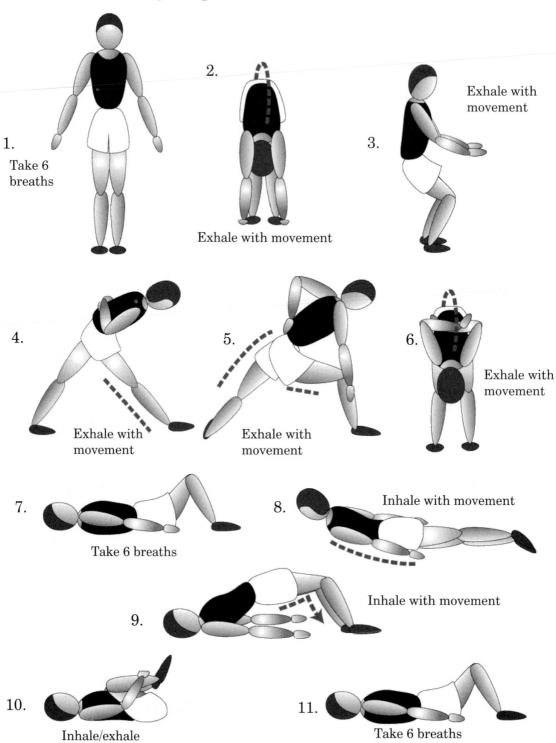

1.

Take 6 breaths

2.

Exhale with movement

3.

Exhale with movement

4.

Exhale with movement

5.

Exhale with movement

6.

Exhale with movement

7.

Take 6 breaths

8.

Inhale with movement

9.

Inhale with movement

10.

Inhale/exhale

11.

Take 6 breaths

Day 5: repeat exercises 2–6 times each

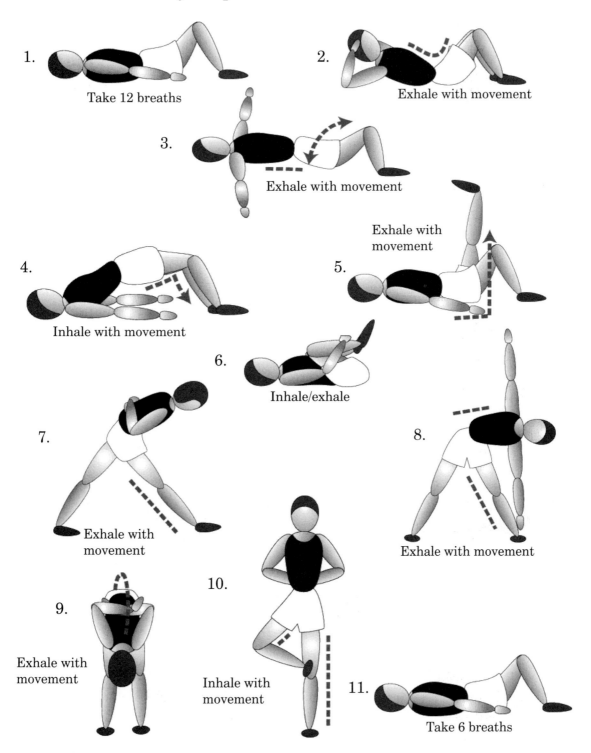

1. Take 12 breaths

2. Exhale with movement

3. Exhale with movement

4. Inhale with movement

5. Exhale with movement

6. Inhale/exhale

7. Exhale with movement

8. Exhale with movement

9. Exhale with movement

10. Inhale with movement

11. Take 6 breaths

Day 6: repeat exercises 2–6 times each

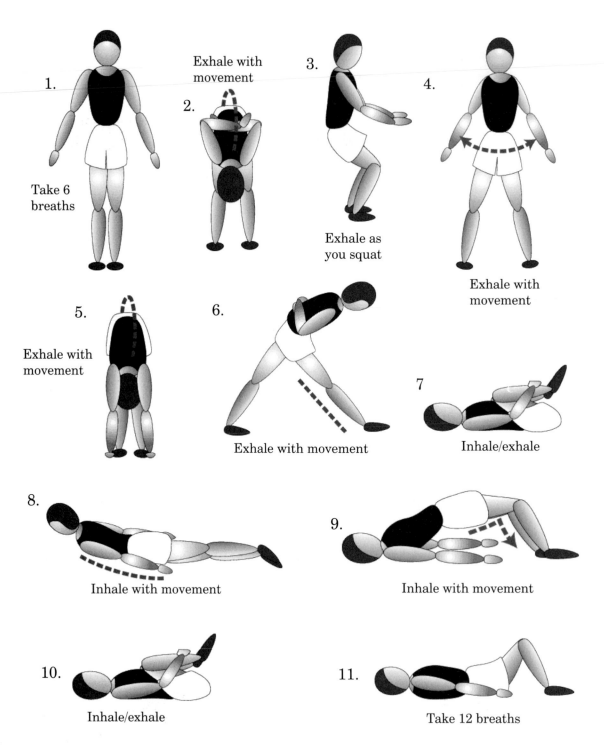

1.

Take 6
breaths

Exhale with
movement

2.

3.

Exhale as
you squat

4.

Exhale with
movement

5.

Exhale with
movement

6.

Exhale with movement

7

Inhale/exhale

8.

Inhale with movement

9.

Inhale with movement

10.

Inhale/exhale

11.

Take 12 breaths

Day 7: repeat exercises 2–6 times each

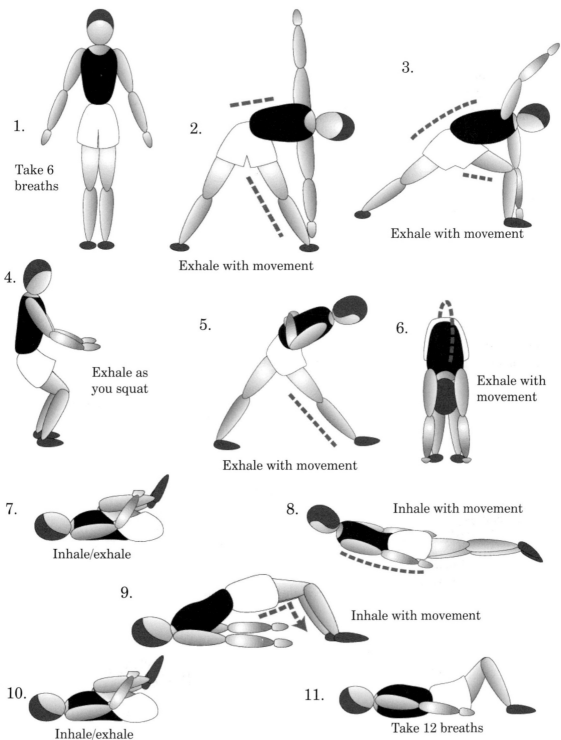

1.

Take 6
breaths

2.

Exhale with movement

3.

Exhale with movement

4.

Exhale as
you squat

5.

Exhale with movement

6.

Exhale with
movement

7.

Inhale/exhale

8.

Inhale with movement

9.

Inhale with movement

10.

Inhale/exhale

11.

Take 12 breaths

Day 8: repeat exercises 2–6 times each

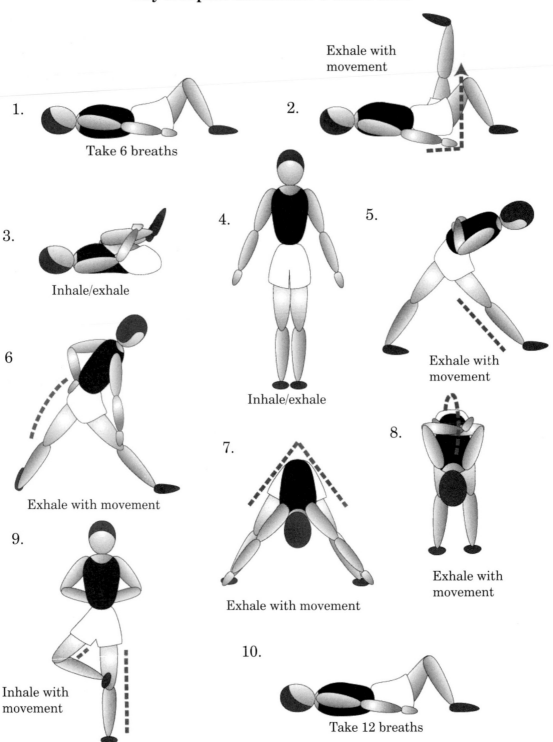

1. Take 6 breaths

2. Exhale with movement

3. Inhale/exhale

4. Inhale/exhale

5. Exhale with movement

6 Exhale with movement

7. Exhale with movement

8. Exhale with movement

9. Inhale with movement

10. Take 12 breaths

Relaxation techniques

Relaxation is an important part of your exercise programme. Relaxation techniques can be learnt very easily. They can be used often and not only when lying on the floor. It is important to work slowly and to breathe correctly. Learn the technique lying on the floor. Lie either with the legs bent or straight. Place a pillow under the knees for support (see *Figure 3.1*).

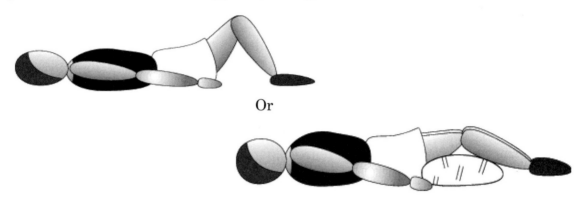

Or

Figure 3.1

Concentrate on the right leg. As you exhale feel the leg become heavy and spread out. Let the muscles relax as you exhale. Do not tighten them first. Do the same with the left leg.

Next relax the pelvic area and abdomen on the exhalation. Check that your legs still feel heavy. Next focus on the spine. Visualise the spine from the neck to the tail. Think about relaxing the muscles that support this area as well as the sides of the back and the shoulders. Remain focused and mentally release the tension.

When your back feels heavy and released move the focus to your right arm and using the exhalation encourage the arm to relax. Do the same with the left arm. Go up through both arms from fingertips to shoulders. Focus on the shoulders making sure they feel heavy. Concentrate on relaxing again.

Finally focus on the face. Release the jaw, the face and the scalp. Now concentrate on your breathing. Every time you breathe out say the word *relax*. Remain in this state of relaxation for as long as possible. When you feel completely relaxed and calm repeat your affirmation several times.

To come out of the state of relaxation gradually stretch the legs and arms. Reintroduce moderate tension into your muscles. Sometimes it is useful to curl up into a ball to come out of the state of relaxation. It may also be useful to use an appropriate compact disc or cassette to listen to.

Final advice

It is impossible to heal the back on a long-term basis unless you view the problem holistically. Think of the mind, body and spirit as a whole. You are not simply a back. You are a body full of bad habits and tensions that have become the norm. Once you begin to programme yourself into the correct way of moving, thinking and exercising you will gradually begin to realise that your body has not been working efficiently and that this has caused the problems with your back. You will realise that you are your body's worst enemy. Therefore you must be prepared to discipline yourself to work with the exercise plans every day. Ensure that you eat a healthy diet that contains at least five servings of fresh fruit or vegetables each day. Make sure you are getting enough vitamins especially the B vitamins in the form of B complex. Be positive about what you are doing and trying to achieve. The brain produces endorphins which make you feel happy and releases more of these when you exercise regularly. Therefore it becomes a circle; regular exercise produces back strength which will help to increase your positive attitude which in turn will benefit your attitude to exercise. Finally, look, feel and think strong, supple back.